Pleural Disease

Editor

JONATHAN PUCHALSKI

CLINICS IN CHEST MEDICINE

www.chestmed.theclinics.com

March 2013 • Volume 34 • Number 1

ELSEVIER

1600 John F. Kennedy Boulevard • Suite 1800 • Philadelphia, Pennsylvania, 19103-2899

http://www.theclinics.com

CLINICS IN CHEST MEDICINE Volume 34, Number 1
March 2013 ISSN 0272-5231, ISBN-13: 978-1-4557-7073-1

Editor: Katie Saunders
Developmental Editor: Donald E. Mumford

Clinics in Chest Medicine (ISSN 0272-5231) is published quarterly by Elsevier Inc., 360 Park Avenue South, New York, NY 10010-1710. Months of issue are March, June, September, and December. Periodicals postage paid at New York, NY and additional mailing offices. Subscription prices are $329.00 per year (domestic individuals), $526.00 per year (domestic institutions), $157.00 per year (domestic students/residents), $361.00 per year (Canadian individuals), $645.00 per year (Canadian institutions), $448.00 per year (international individuals), $645.00 per year (international institutions), and $219.00 per year (international and Canadian students/residents). International air speed delivery is included in all Clinics subscription prices. All prices are subject to change without notice. **POSTMASTER:** Send address changes to Clinics in Chest Medicine, Elsevier Health Sciences Division, Subscription Customer Service, 3251 Riverport Lane, Maryland Heights, MO 63043. **Customer Service: Telephone: 1-800-654-2452** (U.S. and Canada); **1-314-447-8871** (outside U.S. and Canada). **Fax: 1-314-447-8029. E-mail: journalscustomerservice-usa@elsevier.com** (for print support); **journalsonlinesupport-usa@elsevier.com** (for online support).

Reprints. For copies of 100 or more of articles in this publication, please contact the Commercial Reprints Department, Elsevier Inc., 360 Park Avenue South, New York, NY 10010-1710. Tel.: 212-633-3812; Fax: 212-462-1935; E-mail: reprints@elsevier.com.

Clinics in Chest Medicine is covered in *MEDLINE/PubMed (Index Medicus), Current Contents/Clinical Medicine, EMBASE/ Excerpta Medica, Science Citation Index,* and *ISI/BIOMED.*

Printed and bound by CPI Group (UK) Ltd, Croydon, CR0 4YY
Transferred to Digital Printing, 2013

Contributors

EDITOR

JONATHAN PUCHALSKI, MD, MEd
Assistant Professor of Medicine, Director of
Interventional Pulmonology, The Thoracic
Interventional Program, Division of Pulmonary,
Critical Care and Sleep Medicine,
Department of Internal Medicine, Yale
University School of Medicine, New Haven,
Connecticut

AUTHORS

JASON AKULIAN, MD, MPH
Division of Pulmonary and Critical Care
Medicine, The Johns Hopkins University
School of Medicine, Baltimore, Maryland

RAHUL BHATNAGAR, MB ChB, MRCP
Respiratory Specialty Registrar, Respiratory
Research Unit, Southmead Hospital,
Westbury-on-Trym; Clinical Research Fellow,
Academic Respiratory Unit, University of
Bristol, Bristol, United Kingdom

KYLE BRAMLEY, MD
Post-doctoral Fellow, Division of Pulmonary,
Critical Care and Sleep Medicine,
Department of Internal Medicine, Yale
University School of Medicine, New Haven,
Connecticut

HENRI G. COLT, MD, FCCP
Division of Pulmonary and Critical Care
Medicine, Irvine Medical Centre, University of
California, California

FRANK C. DETTERBECK, MD
Professor of Surgery, Department of Thoracic
Surgery, Yale University School of Medicine,
New Haven, Connecticut

CHRISTOPHER T. ERB, MD, PhD
Postdoctoral Fellow, Section of Pulmonary,
Critical Care, and Sleep Medicine, Department
of Internal Medicine, Yale School of Medicine,
New Haven, Connecticut

DAVID FELLER-KOPMAN, MD, FCCP
Director, Bronchoscopy & Interventional
Pulmonology, Division of Pulmonary and
Critical Care Medicine, Associate Professor of
Medicine, Johns Hopkins University School of
Medicine, Baltimore, Maryland

ANDREW R. HAAS, MD, PhD
Assistant Professor, Section of Interventional
Pulmonology and Thoracic Oncology,
Pulmonary, Allergy, and Critical Care Division,
University of Pennsylvania Medical Center,
Philadelphia, Pennsylvania

KELSEY M. JOHNSON, PA-C
Yale Thoracic Interventional Program, Smilow
Cancer Hospital at Yale-New Haven Hospital,
New Haven, Connecticut

ANTHONY W. KIM, MD
Assistant Professor of Medicine, Thoracic
Surgery, Thoracic Oncology Program, Smilow
Cancer Hospital at Yale-New Haven Hospital,
Yale School of Medicine, New Haven,
Connecticut

HANS J. LEE, MD
Virginia Commonwealth University Medical
Center, Richmond, Virginia

PYNG LEE, MD, FCCP
Division of Respiratory and Critical Care
Medicine, Department of Medicine, Associate
Professor, Yong Loo Lin Medical School,
National University Hospital, National
University of Singapore, Singapore

RICHARD W. LIGHT, MD
Division of Allergy/Pulmonary/Critical Care,
Vanderbilt University Medical Center,
Professor of Medicine, Vanderbilt University,
Nashville, Tennessee

KAMRAN MAHMOOD, MD, MPH
Division of Pulmonary, Allergy and Critical Care
Medicine, Department of Medicine, Duke
University Medical Center, Durham, North
Carolina

NICK A. MASKELL, DM, FRCP
Reader in Respiratory Medicine, Academic
Respiratory Unit, University of Bristol;
Consultant Respiratory Physician, North
Bristol Lung Unit, Southmead Hospital,
Westbury-on-Trym, Bristol, United Kingdom

GAETANE MICHAUD, MD, FCCP, FRCPC
New Haven, Connecticut

RENELLE MYERS, MD, FRCPC
Winnipeg, Manitoba, Canada

JOSÉ M. PORCEL, MD, FCCP, FACP
Professor of Medicine, University of Lleida;
Chief, Department of Internal Medicine, Arnau

de Vilanova University Hospital; Head, Pleural
Diseases Unit, Biomedical Research Institute
of Lleida, Lleida, Spain

JONATHAN T. PUCHALSKI, MD, MEd
Assistant Professor of Medicine, Director of
Interventional Pulmonology, The Thoracic
Interventional Program, Division of Pulmonary,
Critical Care and Sleep Medicine, Department
of Internal Medicine, Yale University School of
Medicine, New Haven, Connecticut

ASHUTOSH SACHDEVA, MBBS
University of Maryland Medical Center,
Baltimore, Maryland

RAY WESLEY SHEPHERD, MD
Virginia Commonwealth University Medical
Center, Richmond, Virginia

DANIEL H. STERMAN, MD
Associate Professor of Medicine and Surgery,
Chief, Section of Interventional Pulmonology
and Thoracic Oncology, Pulmonary, Allergy,
and Critical Care Division, University of
Pennsylvania Medical Center, Philadelphia,
Pennsylvania

MOMEN M. WAHIDI, MD, MBA
Division of Pulmonary, Allergy and Critical Care
Medicine, Department of Medicine, Duke
University Medical Center, Durham,
North Carolina

LONNY YARMUS, DO
Division of Pulmonary and Critical Care
Medicine, Assistant Professor of Medicine, The
Johns Hopkins University School of Medicine,
Baltimore, Maryland

Contents

SECTION I: OBTAINING PLEURAL FLUID

Thoracentesis is one of the most common medical procedures performed today. With the advent of thoracic ultrasound, thoracentesis has been enhanced with additional preprocedural, intraprocedural, and postprocedural information. The authors review modern-day thoracentesis and the use of ultrasonography. Nearly 200,000 thoracenteses are performed among 1.5 million patients with pleural effusion each year. A solid foundation in didactic knowledge and procedural proficiency is important to avoid unwanted complications. Ultrasound has become an indispensable tool to guide performance of thoracentesis. Ultrasonography for this purpose has several advantages. The authors provide a contemporary review on thoracentesis and the use of ultrasonography.

Pleural disease is commonly encountered by the chest physician. Evaluation of pleural disease typically begins with thoracentesis and pleural fluid analysis. With improvements in minimally invasive procedures, imaging, and the use of pleural manometry, a more complete understanding of lung, pleural, and chest wall physiology is possible. The improved knowledge of pleural physiology can help the clinician in clinical decision making, as well as the diagnosis and treatment of pleural disease. This article reviews pleural physiology and summarizes the relevant data supporting the use of ultrasound and manometry in the evaluation and treatment of pleural disease.

SECTION II: ANALYZING PLEURAL FLUID

The Light criteria serve as a good starting point in the separation of transudates from exudates. The Light criteria misclassify about 25% of transudates as exudates, and most of these patients are on diuretics. If a patient is thought likely to have a disease that produces a transudative pleural effusion but the Light criteria suggest an exudate by only a small margin, the serum–pleural fluid protein gradient should be examined.

CLINICS IN CHEST MEDICINE

DOWNLOAD
Free App!

Review Articles
THE CLINICS

NOW AVAILABLE FOR YOUR iPhone and iPad

Preface

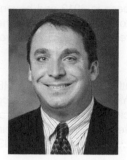

Jonathan Puchalski, MD, MEd
Editor

Pleural diseases affect over a million individuals annually, and physicians in most subspecialties encounter pleural effusions. This issue of *Clinics in Chest Medicine* aims to succinctly define what is, in my opinion, critical to know for clinical practice in 2013. I asked Dr Light to give us insight into what he has learned since the establishment of Light's criteria 40 years ago, and I invite you to relive his experiences and embrace the "take-home points" from his amazing career.

Although a thoracentesis can be performed by reviewing radiographs and performing an appropriate physical examination, the widespread use and portability of ultrasound (US) has changed practice in many centers. As US becomes "pocket-sized," it makes sense to apply US for most pleural interventions, and I very strongly encourage anybody who does not know how to perform a basic thoracic US to take the relatively short amount of time required to learn. Although we each have different learning thresholds, US can readily identify the best location in which to perform the thoracentesis and it can give an idea about how complex the effusion may be. The first article highlights the practical advantages of US and it becomes clear that US enables a simple means of providing safe, evidence-based practice.

A thorough understanding of pleural physiology allows us to understand much about the underlying causes of pleural effusions, but also enables us to determine which pneumothoraces do not require chest tubes or which pleural diseases require decortication. The second article provides an excellent description from experts in the field. I call your attention to the images, which show how this can easily be performed at the bedside without complex adaptors or equipment.

The next two articles allow us to understand what has transpired over the past four decades in determining groups of effusions and elucidating causes. Light's criteria remain extremely useful in assessing etiologies of effusions, while other biomarkers have emerged to more specifically identify causes. Although the possibilities of many complex molecules may seem overwhelming, these reviews offer a manageable approach to defining pleural disease into transudates, exudates, and beyond.

Article five provides an overview of those effusions that result from intra-abdominal processes. Although heart failure, malignancy, and pneumonia are prominent causes of effusions, intricate connections enable fluid to pass in one direction from the abdomen into the pleural space. Some of the most fascinating causes of pleural disease arise from below the diaphragm.

The next three articles discuss the management of complex pleural effusions and help to determine nonsurgical means of draining effusions not amenable to thoracentesis. Instillation of various agents into the pleural space may avert the need for surgical intervention in many patients, as shown in the sixth article. The following article addresses the common questions of "How big?" and "What type?" of chest tubes are needed for these complex effusions and other disease processes. Article eight gives a step-by-step overview of tunneled pleural catheter placement and focuses on the practical aspects of these indwelling chest tubes. These topics are essential for anybody with an interest in pleural disease.

Clin Chest Med 34 (2013) ix–x
http://dx.doi.org/10.1016/j.ccm.2013.01.001
0272-5231/13/$ – see front matter © 2013 Published by Elsevier Inc.

The goal of the next articles is to discuss thoracoscopy and to help provide a practical understanding of differences between the medical and surgical endoscopic evaluation of the pleural space. Through the input of world-renowned medical and surgical physicians, I hope these perspectives clarify when one technique may be more useful than the other.

Finally, this edition of *Clinics in Chest Medicine* covers primary pleural tumors. Article 11 focuses on mesothelioma, while article 12 gives a rare overview of other tumors that may be encountered in the pleural space. The pictures take us into the pleural cavity for an up-to-date depiction of what happens when cancer develops in this unique space.

I hope you enjoy this exciting topic and find that the concepts discussed herein enhance your approach to pleural disease is 2013 and beyond. I'm forever indebted to my mentors for their teaching and am inspired by my children every day.

Jonathan Puchalski, MD, MEd
Interventional Pulmonology
The Thoracic Interventional Program
Yale University School of Medicine
New Haven, CT 06510, USA

E-mail address:
Jonathan.puchalski@yale.edu

Prologue
What I Have Learned in the Past 40 Years

In this special edition of *Clinics in Chest Medicine*, I was asked to write a prologue about my career and highlight my educational opportunities en route to becoming a Professor of Medicine at Vanderbilt University. I have learned many things in the past 40 years since the publications of the Light criteria for pleural effusions. I have learned what it takes to be successful. I think that successful researchers have several attributes. (1) They are organized. They do not waste time looking for things or repeating things. (2) They are persistent. If a grant or a manuscript gets rejected, they keep trying. (3) In their research, they create win-win situations. If the person you need to cooperate on a research project gets nothing for cooperating, they probably will not do much. (4) They take advantage of opportunities in their present location. For example, when I moved to Saint Thomas Hospital in Nashville, Tennessee, many patients were undergoing coronary artery bypass graft surgery (CABG). I wrote several articles on post-CABG pleural effusions to optimize this opportunity. (5) They are happy and part of this is sleeping with the right person!

Pleural disease is more popular in countries other than the United States. I am currently invited to give more lectures in foreign countries than in the United States. I attribute this to the emphasis at national pulmonary conferences in other countries being on clinical problems rather than basic mechanisms.

Funding for pleural research is poor. The National Institutes of Health funds few grants whose main focus is pleural disease. Pharmaceutical companies are hesitant to fund research on pleural disease. For example, we have shown that intrapleural transforming growth factor β (TGF β) in animals produces a faster and better pleurodesis than talc or the tetracycline compounds. However, we have been unable to induce any pharmaceutical company to study TGF β in humans. As another example, the correct dose and the length of action of tissue plasminogen activator (tPA) for the treatment of complicated parapneumonic effusions is unknown. However, the company that produces tPA does not support animal studies to answer these questions.

There are many unanswered questions concerning pleural disease. Are malignant effusions best treated with indwelling catheters or by the induction of pleurodesis with agents injected into the pleural space? Are patients with complicated parapneumonic effusions best treated with the combination of tPA and DNase or with thoracoscopy? Is spontaneous pneumothorax best treated with medical thoracoscopy or with video-assisted thoracic surgery?

If I had to do it over it over again, I would not change much. I have been lucky throughout my career. An example of this luck is that the first article I wrote was on the Light criteria. Of all the articles that I have written, this was the simplest, but it made me the most famous. The institutions that I have worked at have all been good places to work. The foreign researchers who worked with me on pleural disease served as a constant source of stimulation.

There are a few things that I would change. I would have started animal research earlier: my first article involving animal research was in 1993. It is a lot easier to recruit animals than humans to participate in research projects. I would have focused more on pleural disease; I spent much time studying exercise and anxiety and depression in chronic obstructive pulmonary disease and virtually no one knows that I ever did any research in these areas. I would not have become the Associate Chief of Staff at the Veterans' Affairs Hospital in Long Beach, California. In this position, I spent many hours reviewing other people's grants and thought that my efforts in this capacity decreased my productivity in pulmonary research.

In summary, I have enjoyed my career and am excited by ongoing developments in pleural disease. I hope that funding improves but encourage anyone, at any stage of their career, to persist in their efforts and maximize the opportunities available from the resources surrounding them.

Richard W. Light, MD
Professor of Medicine, Vanderbilt University
Division of Allergy/Pulmonary/Critical Care
Vanderbilt University Medical Center
Vanderbilt University, 1161 21st Avenue South
Nashville, TN 37232, USA

E-mail address:
Rlight98@yahoo.com

Clin Chest Med 34 (2013) xi
http://dx.doi.org/10.1016/j.ccm.2013.01.002
0272-5231/13/$ – see front matter © 2013 Published by Elsevier Inc.

Thoracentesis and Thoracic Ultrasound: State of the Art in 2013

Ashutosh Sachdeva, MBBS[a], Ray Wesley Shepherd, MD[b],
Hans J. Lee, MD[b],*

KEYWORDS

- Thoracentesis • Thoracic ultrasound • Pleural effusion

KEY POINTS

- Thoracentesis is an invaluable tool for assessing pleural disease.
- The use of ultrasonography by trained professionals has enhanced this procedure's safety and feasibility.
- Routine ultrasonography enhances preprocedural, intraprocedural, and postprocedural assessment of the pleural space.
- As equipment becomes more available and portable, its use is anticipated to grow and possibly become the standard of care.

DIAGNOSTIC AND THERAPEUTIC THORACENTESIS

The clinical or radiological recognition of a pleural effusion suggests an abnormal pathophysiological state resulting in an imbalance between absorption and production of fluid in the pleural space.[1–7] Thoracentesis is often divided into 2 categories, namely, diagnostic aspiration and therapeutic removal. Diagnostic thoracentesis is performed to obtain a small volume of fluid (50–100 mL) for the purpose of analysis, which is accomplished with a single percutaneous needle aspiration.

A therapeutic thoracentesis is performed to relieve symptoms, such as dyspnea, to relieve hemodynamic compromise or to evacuate the pleural space of infection.[8] The therapeutic thoracentesis is normally accomplished using a temporary catheter that is removed at the end of volume removal. These categorizations are often blurred because an initial aspiration may be done to provide both analysis and relief of symptoms. It would be reasonable to consider maximal removal of pleural effusion if an aspiration is already occurring. With this mindset, a diagnostic thoracentesis would only be performed if a therapeutic aspiration were not safe, feasible, or under other unusual circumstances.

Indications and Complications

There are no absolute contraindications to performing a diagnostic thoracentesis. Risks and benefits should be carefully considered when performing thoracentesis in patients with relative contraindications, such as a bleeding diathesis or those on anticoagulation therapy. It is debated if commonly measured parameters, including prothrombin time and activated partial thromboplastin time, alone predict the risk of bleeding complications, although thrombocytopenia along with renal dysfunction (serum creatinine >6 mg/dL) likely portends higher risks.[9,10] Some investigators have suggested the use of a structured questionnaire to generate a bleeding score for predicting complications before invasive procedures.[11] Furthermore, it is

The authors have nothing to disclose.
Disclosures: None.
[a] University of Maryland Medical Center, 110 South Paca Street, 2nd Floor, Baltimore, MD 210, USA; [b] Virginia Commonwealth University Medical Center, PO BOX 980050, Richmond, VA 23298-0050, USA
* Corresponding author. Virginia Commonwealth University Medical Center, PO BOX 980050, Richmond, VA 23298-0050.
E-mail address: snah74@hotmail.com

chestmed.theclinics.com

unclear if concurrent therapy with clopidogrel or similar classes of drugs alters the risk of bleeding complications. Thromboelastography has been shown to be a better assay for detecting mild coagulation abnormalities associated with an increased risk of bleeding in a select group of patients undergoing renal biopsies, although its utility in thoracentesis has not been studied.[12] Other tests measuring platelet function have been used for patients undergoing coronary artery bypass graft but have not been investigated in patients on clopidogrel undergoing thoracentesis.[13]

Infectious complications related to thoracentesis are rare. In a study addressing this specifically, Cervini and colleagues[14] reported no infections despite a large number of thoracenteses performed. However, one must be cognizant of placing a needle or catheter through infected subcutaneous tissue or skin into the sterile pleural space.

Pneumothorax is a potential serious complication associated with thoracentesis and may contribute to morbidity.[4,15] The rates of pneumothorax while using ultrasound (US) have ranged from 1.3% to 6.7%.[15–17] The incidence of pneumothorax without the use of US has been reported with rates varying between 4% and 30%.[3,18,19] A pneumothorax related to thoracentesis may occur in 3 different scenarios: (1) atmospheric air introduction with the catheter removal or aspiration of fluid; (2) needle injury to the visceral pleura, permitting air to enter from the alveoli; and (3) rapid decrease in pleural pressure from aspiration resulting in visceral pleura rupture.[2,20]

Because of the concern for pneumothorax, there were previously concerns about the safety of thoracentesis in patients on mechanical ventilation. However, studies have demonstrated that the risk of complication is no higher in patients requiring ventilation than in nonmechanically ventilated patients. In one of the largest series of thoracentesis using US on mechanically ventilated patients, only 3 out of 232 (1.3%) had a pneumothorax, none had tension physiology, and only 1 (0.004%) required chest tube placement.[21] In this study, medical residents under attending supervision performed all needle insertions. Other investigators have cited the theoretical risk of a bronchopleural fistula (BPF) after a pneumothorax.[20] The use of small-gauge needles and US make BPF a very uncommon complication from diagnostic thoracentesis.

Other reported complications include splenic laceration, abdominal hemorrhage, intrathoracic hemorrhage, sheared off catheter, tumor seeding of the needle tract, hemothorax, pneumohemothorax, anxiety, and site pain.[3,18,22–26]

Therapeutic thoracentesis has the additional complications of reexpansion pulmonary edema, hypovolemia, and hypoxemia.[27,28] It is thought that these complications are caused by large volumes of pleural fluid being removed in a single setting. Reexpansion pulmonary edema after thoracentesis represents a potentially life-threatening complication with a mortality rate as high as 20%.[29] Fortunately, the occurrence of reexpansion pulmonary edema is rare (0.2%–0.5%).[30,31] Some experts have recommend maximal removal of 1.0 to 1.5 L to avoid this complication[32]; however, the more pertinent factor may be avoiding a decrease in end-expiratory pleural pressure less than −20 cm H_2O. By using manometry, larger volumes have been removed safely while avoiding a more negative pleural pressure.[30,33,34] Also, symptoms of chest discomfort have been associated with a decrease pleural pressure less than −20 cm H_2O, and an inverse relationship was found with coughing during volume removal.[35]

Anatomic Considerations

Intercostal spaces (ICS) are an important access portal for entering the pleural space for thoracentesis and chest tube insertion. US-assisted thoracentesis requires familiarization of the traditional anatomic landmarks (ie, course of neurovascular bundle at the inferior aspect of rib in the subcostal groove) but also variability in the course of the intercostal artery (ICA), especially in elderly patients (**Fig. 1**).[36–38] The collateral ICA that usually runs on the superior border of inferior rib can be lacerated during thoracic procedures with the needle or during catheter insertion.[39] Two different studies have demonstrated that the ICA

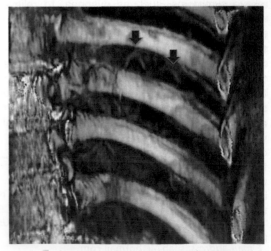

Fig. 1. Tortuous course of intercostal artery in an elderly individual (*bold arrows*).

is more exposed in the center of the interspace in positions more posteriorly. Furthermore, studies have demonstrated that the ICA may be 20% of the way down into the ICS even as far laterally as the midaxillary line.[38,40] Therefore, unless fluid is loculated posteriorly, this approach should be reconsidered.[38,41] The British Thoracic Society's guidelines recommend the insertion of the needle in the triangle of safety (anterior border of latissimus dorsi, the lateral border of pectoralis major, and a horizontal line lateral at the level of the nipple) to avoid the ICA. However, an approach 9 to 10 cm lateral to the spine in the posterior axillary line is equally acceptable, especially in patients sitting upright.[32]

Procedural Technique

Adequate positioning of patients is important to safely perform thoracentesis. Patients may be more comfortable while sitting on the edge of the bed with their arms and head resting on one or more pillows on a table and footstool supporting the feet. For patients unable to sit, a needle puncture may be attempted in the midaxillary line with the head of the bed maximally elevated and the arm positioned above the shoulders. Alternatively, the procedure can be performed with patients in the lateral decubitus position with the effusion side nondependent. This position may be an optimal position for patients unable to follow instructions or who are too ill to support sitting upright.

Thoracentesis is performed under aseptic precautions. Once the site is properly marked using US, attention is then directed to local anesthesia. Given that the parietal pleura, rib periosteum, and epidermal nerve endings are the most sensitive area for pain during thoracentesis, lidocaine should be applied to these areas. The finder needle is used to penetrate the skin and subcutaneous tissue while continuously aspirating until fluid is aspirated. If the needle contacts a rib, an anesthetic may be injected and the needle repositioned superior to the rib. After fluid is obtained, the finder needle may be retracted until aspiration stops. This location is close to the parietal pleural and can then be anesthetized generously, after which the seeker needle is withdrawn. A catheter over a placement needle is then advanced, following the same track into the pleural space with continued manual aspiration. A small stab incision may be necessary to prevent kinking of the catheter as it enters the subcutaneous tissue. The catheter is advanced while the needle is kept still with the elbow holding the aspiration syringe relatively fixed to the body. On fluid retrieval, the catheter is advanced into the pleural

space and the needle removed. The catheter is then attached to a drainage system. The use of a vacuum bottle drainage system has been associated with a higher risk for pneumothorax, and manual aspiration is preferred.[42] There may be several variations of this technique depending on operator experience and the type of commercial catheter used.

Specimen Handling

Diagnostic thoracentesis requires approximately 50 mL of pleural fluid. Common tests performed on pleural fluid include cell count with differential, pH, total protein, lactate dehydrogenase, glucose, gram stain and culture, and cytology. Additional tests (**Table 1**) include pleural fluid hematocrit, albumin, brain natriuretic peptide, adenosine deaminase, triglycerides, cholesterol, amylase, and mycobacterial or fungal cultures, depending on the clinical scenario. For cell count and differential, the fluid should be placed in EDTA-treated tubes if the syringe was not initially heparinized because fluid collected in tubes without anticoagulants can give inaccurate numbers.[43] Fluid pH should be measured with a blood gas machine whenever a parapneumonic effusion or malignancy is suspected.[44] Collection of pleural fluid for the measurement of pH warrants careful attention because admixture of air, lidocaine, or heparin with pleural fluid alters the measured pH.[45,46] If analyzed expeditiously, it is not necessary to place samples on ice because the pH of a sample at room temperature does not change significantly during the first hour following thoracentesis.[47]

In addition to the previously mentioned tests, fluid may be sent separately for cytologic preparation. One should consult with their institutional

Table 1		
Additional tests on pleural fluid		
Tests	**Clinical Scenario**	
Hematocrit	Hemothorax	
Albumin	Gradient helpful in differentiating transudate vs exudate	
BNP level	CHF	
Adenosine deaminase	Tuberculosis	
Triglyceride	Chylothorax	
Cholesterol	Pseudochylothorax, rheumatoid arthritis, chronic pleuritis	

Abbreviations: BNP, brain natriuretic peptide; CHF, congestive heart failure.

pathologists to determine the optimal means of delivering fluid for analysis; but typically fluid may be analyzed by thin preparations, cytospin, cell blocks, and other techniques. It is generally recommended that both cell blocks and smears be used in evaluating all fluids submitted to the cytology laboratory.[48–51] In addition to processing the sample, other factors, such as type of tumor, associated other diagnosis (heart failure, pulmonary emboli, pneumonia, lymphatic obstruction, or hypoproteinemia), and tumor burden, among others, may alter the diagnostic yield.[52] For the purposes of evaluating a malignant pleural effusion, only 50 to 60 mL of fluid is required because larger volumes do not significantly increase the yield of pleural fluid cytology.[53,54] On the other hand, analyzing less volume seems to reduce the diagnostic yield for pleural malignancy.[55]

Role of Follow-up Imaging

A routine chest radiograph after thoracentesis is not required for most asymptomatic and nonventilated patients.[56,57] This point was best illustrated by a prospective study whereby, of the 488 asymptomatic patients, only one patient was found to have pneumothorax on a postthoracentesis radiograph.[58] If, however, the primary purpose for a postprocedural radiograph is to assess lung expansion and assess for potential lung entrapment, trapped lung, and future therapeutic decision making, then obtaining a plain radiograph in asymptomatic patients is reasonable. Alternatives to a postprocedural radiograph may include the use of US to detect complications and to determine the presence of remaining fluid. On the other hand, a manometer attached to the thoracentesis catheter can provide information regarding the expandability of the lung.

Pleural US

US has been used in the medical field for more than 50 years.[59] Nonradiology specialties are currently using US in various applications, including emergency medicine, endocrinology, cardiology, surgery, and obstetrics. It has been only within the past decade that US has gained popularity by pulmonologists. This popularity may have been facilitated by decreasing costs, increasing portability, and increasing education regarding the technology.

The basic hardware requirements include a transducer, US machine, and image storage capacity. The transducer should have a probe that will fit between the intercostal space; typically, this is the same as the abdominal probe and distinct from a vascular and other probes. The frequency of the US probe should be 3.5 to 5.0

MHz.[60] Lower-frequency US have better penetration but lower image resolution, whereas higher-frequency US provides better images but decreases visualization of deeper structures. The frequency within 3.5 to 5.0 MHz allows for a balance of depth and clarity for pleural imaging. Of course, structures such as the ribs prevent US waves from traversing the tissue and result in artifacts.

Aside from the size and portability of the US machine, as well as use of specified probes, image storage and Doppler capabilities may be considered. Image storage and labeling are essential when billing for the use of US to guide the thoracentesis. Thoracentesis uses CPT code 32421 or 32422, whereas US is an add-on code (76942–26). Although Doppler is not necessary, in select cases, it can image aberrant vessels that prohibit a selected procedural target point.[61]

In addition to hardware, thoracic US requires skills to perform and interpret pleural US. With appropriate training, this can be accomplished. A prospective study comparing the diagnostic accuracy of pulmonologists with radiologists in identifying pleural effusions was 99.6% correct and garnered no false positives.[62] Other studies have supported the use of US by nonradiologists in accurately interpreting findings of hemoperitoneum and performing basic general US examinations in intensive care units.[63,64] Recognizing the importance of US for performing thoracentesis, the current American College of Graduate Medical Education program requirements mandate pulmonary/critical care fellowship programs to provide education on US techniques to perform thoracentesis.[65,66] In some medical schools, portable US devices are now a part of their physical examination curriculum.[67]

Although US can access up to 70% of the pleural surface, there remain some areas that are limited on US visualization because of the bony thoracic cage.[68] Furthermore, because US waves do not travel through an air medium, certain conditions with bullae or extensive subcutaneous air may hamper US imaging of the pleural surface. The air barrier may also, at times, limit the visualization of the normal lung parenchyma. Another potential limitation is the variable individual operator skills and experience to obtain/interpret images correctly. The American College of Chest Physicians/Société de Réanimation de Langue Française have published guidelines for US competence in pulmonary/critical care.[69]

Preprocedural and Intraprocedural US

US may be useful before, during, and after the thoracentesis (**Table 2**).

Table 2	
Advantages of US-guided thoracentesis	
Preprocedure	Evaluate patient at bedside immediately before procedure
	Evaluate quantity of pleural effusion
	Assess potential procedural difficulties
	Assess differential diagnosis based on US appearance
Intraprocedure	Assess best entry point
	Place needle or catheter in real time
	Avoid injury to other structures
Postprocedure	Evaluate for pneumothorax
	Evaluate extent of remaining fluid

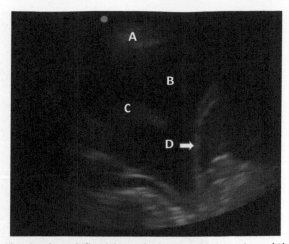

Fig. 2. Pleural fluid boundaries on US imaging. (A) Chest wall, (B) pleural effusion, (C) atelectatic lung, (D) diaphragm.

The key advantages of US with preprocedural assessment of the pleural space include a point-of-care evaluation, assessment of potential anatomic procedural difficulties, generating differential diagnoses, and marking the best site of entry. US has shown to be more sensitive and accurate compared with lateral decubitus radiography in detecting pleural effusions.[66,70] In a prospective study, bedside US improved the puncture site selection in up to 54% of the patients when physicians were unable to locate a puncture site by physical examination. Also, in the same study, US prevented potential accidental organ puncture in 10% of all cases.[71] It is important to note that the benefit of US site selection in decreasing pneumothoraces occurs with only real-time needle puncture or immediate preprocedure marking (patient in same position/location). Notably, US marking of the effusion to perform the thoracentesis at a later time or location does not reduce iatrogenic pneumothoraces.[66,72]

Preprocedural identification of adhesions and complex loculations may predict successful pleural space access for thoracentesis or other pleural procedures. In a retrospective study, US characteristics of empyema predicted the success of drainage with a complex or septated sonographic pattern having less success.[73] Furthermore, thoracic US before medical thoracoscopy improved pleural access and predicted fibrous septations.[74] **Figs. 2–4** demonstrate different US patterns seen in pleural effusions.

Postprocedure US

There are several advantages of using US after a pleural procedure such as thoracentesis. It allows for an immediate evaluation of the volume and character of effusion remaining, facilitating medical decision making as to whether more needs removed. Postprocedural bedside US also allows the proceduralist to immediately manage complications, such as pneumothorax.

The first reported US findings of pneumothorax were described in 1986 on a horse.[75] Today, US has been shown to be more sensitive than chest radiograph for the detection of a pneumothorax.[76,77] In a study comparing computed tomography (CT) with US, US detected 92% of pneumothoraces seen on CT scan.[76,78] In another study, pleural US demonstrated superiority over chest radiographs in detecting residual pneumothorax following a drainage procedure.[79] All pneumothoraces detected on US resulted in therapeutic intervention. Using US, the lack of lung sliding and/or the absence of B lines have been described by Lichenstein and colleagues[80] as strong indicators of pneumothorax. The presence of B lines and lung sliding rules out a pneumothorax (negative predictive value 100%).[81] Less reliable signs that have been described for US detection of pneumothorax include lung point (100% specificity; estimates size of pneumothorax) and lung pulse (rules out pneumothorax).[81,82]

US can also be used to detect pulmonary edema and may be useful to confirm suspicion of reexpansion pulmonary edema. US B lines (comet-tail artifact, lung rockets) are the US equivalent of Kerley lines on chest radiograph (97% sensitivity, 95% specificity).[83,84] They appear as vertical narrow lines arising from the pleural line to the edge of the US screen.[85]

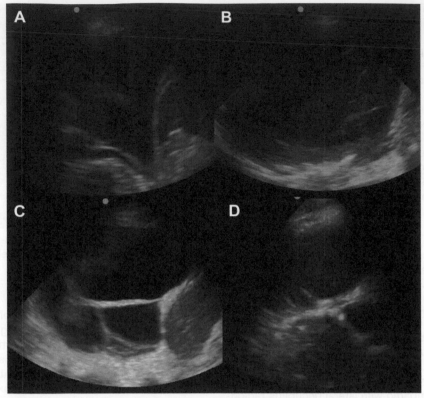

Fig. 3. US patterns of pleural effusion. (*A*) Anechoic, simple, (*B*) complex nonseptated, (*C*) complex septated, (*D*) homogenous echogenic.

Pleural Procedural Service

Specialized services in pleural procedures and disease management have recently become more popular with the expanding number of pleural procedures available to physicians and the accessibility of US.[86,87] In addition, there is a growing number of patients presenting with pleural disease, caused by both infectious and malignant causes.[87–91] A successful procedural unit may facilitate a rapid diagnosis and treatment of pleural disease. In cases of pleural infections, an early diagnosis may make a significant difference in a patient's outcome. Furthermore, the development of a dedicated service provides the opportunity for research in pleural disease.[92] Finally, a dedicated pleural procedural service provides a training environment for education. Frequent repetition with experienced senior supervision may permit learning of thoracic US and thoracentesis skills.

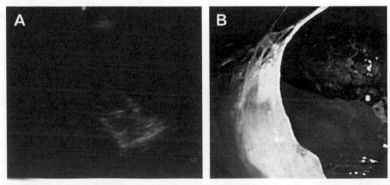

Fig. 4. Confirmation of US images and thoracoscopy. (*A*) US image of pleural effusion with adhesion. (*B*) Same adhesion band visualized on pleuroscopy.

A potential criticism to a dedicated thoracentesis procedural service is that it decreases the number of routine thoracentesis performed by other, perhaps qualified, individuals. Most pulmonologists are experienced with thoracentesis; but when additional skills are added, such as US, manometry, and complication management (tube thoracostomy), the number of qualified pulmonologists decreases. In a retrospective series examining complications before and after instituting a thoracentesis service, there was a significant and dramatic decrease in complications by using a select group of pulmonologists to perform all the thoracentesis at a single institution.[62]

SUMMARY

Thoracentesis is an invaluable tool for assessing pleural disease. The use of US by trained professionals has enhanced this procedure's safety and feasibility. Routine US enhances the preprocedural, intraprocedural, and postprocedural assessment of the pleural space. As equipment becomes more available and portable, its use is anticipated to grow and possibly become the standard of care.

REFERENCES

1. Owings MF, Kozak LJ. Ambulatory and inpatient procedures in the United States, 1996. Vital Health Stat 13 1998;(139):1–119.
2. Light RW, editor. Pleural diseases. 5th edition. Philadelphia: Lippincott, Williams & Wilkins; 2007.
3. Seneff MG, Corwin RW, Gold LH, et al. Complications associated with thoracentesis. Chest 1986;90:97–100.
4. Despars JA, Sassoon CS, Light RW. Significance of iatrogenic pneumothoraces. Chest 1994;105:1147–50.
5. Colt HG, Brewer N, Barbur E. Evaluation of patient-related and procedure-related factors contributing to pneumothorax following thoracentesis. Chest 1999;116:134–8.
6. Feller-Kopman D. Ultrasound-guided thoracentesis. Chest 2006;129:1709–14.
7. Sahn SA. State of the art. The Pleura. Am Rev Respir Dis 1988;138:184–234.
8. Estenne M, Yernault JC, De Troyer A. Mechanisms of relief of dyspnea after thoracentesis in patients with large effusions. Am J Med 1983;74:813–9.
9. Chee YL, Greaves M. Role of coagulation testing in predicting bleeding risk. Hematol J 2003;4:373–8.
10. McVay PA, Toy PT. Lack of increased bleeding after paracentesis and thoracentesis in patients with mild coagulation abnormalities. Transfusion 1991;31:164–71.
11. Watson HG, Greaves M. Can we predict bleeding? Semin Thromb Hemost 2008;34:97–103.
12. Davis CL, Chandler WL. Thromboelastography for the prediction of bleeding after transplant renal biopsy. J Am Soc Nephrol 1995;6:1250–5.
13. Mahla E, Suarez TA, Bliden KP, et al. Platelet function measurement-based strategy to reduce bleeding and waiting time in clopidogrel-treated patients undergoing coronary artery bypass graft surgery: the timing based on platelet function strategy to reduce clopidogrel-associated bleeding related to CABG (TARGET-CABG) study. Circ Cardiovasc Interv 2012;5:261–9.
14. Cervini P, Hesley GK, Thompson RL, et al. Incidence of infectious complications after an ultrasound-guided intervention. Am J Roentgenol 2010;195:846–50.
15. Sassoon CS, Light RW, O'Hara VS, et al. Iatrogenic pneumothorax: etiology and morbidity. Results of a Department of Veterans Affairs cooperative study. Respiration 1992;59:215–20.
16. Barnes TW, Morgenthaler TI, Olson EF, et al. Sonographically guided thoracentesis and rate of pneumothorax. J Clin Ultrasound 2005;33:442–6.
17. Gervais DA, Petersein A, Lee MJ, et al. US-guided thoracentesis: requirement for postprocedure chest radiography in patients who receive mechanical ventilation versus patients who breathe spontaneously. Radiology 1997;204:503–6.
18. Collins TR, Sahn SA. Thoracentesis. Clinical value, complications, technical problems, and patient experience. Chest 1986;91:817–22.
19. Grogan DR, Irwin RS, Channick R, et al. Complications associated with thoracentesis. A prospective, randomized study comparing three different methods. Arch Intern Med 1990;150:873–7.
20. Heidecker J, Huggins JT, Sahn SA, et al. Pathophysiology of pneumothorax following ultrasound-guided thoracentesis. Chest 2006;130:1173–84.
21. Mayo PH, Goltz HR, Tafreshi M, et al. Safety of ultrasound-guided thoracentesis in patients receiving mechanical ventilation. Chest 2004;125:1059–61.
22. Braveny I, Machka K. Delayed iatrogenic rupture of the spleen. Lancet 1980;2:752–3.
23. Heffner JE, Sahn SA. Abdominal hemorrhage after perforation of a diaphragmatic artery during thoracentesis. Arch Intern Med 1981;141:1238.
24. Carney M, Ravin CE. Intercostal artery laceration during thoracentesis. Increased risk in elderly patients. Chest 1979;75:520–2.
25. Sue DY, Lam K. Retention of catheter fragment after thoracentesis. Postgrad Med 1982;72:101–6.
26. Agurlar-Torres FG, Schlueter DP, Perlman L, et al. Subcutaneous implantation of an adenocarcinoma following thoracentesis. Wis Med J 1977;76:19–21.
27. Trapnell DH, Thurston JB. Unilateral pulmonary edema after pleural aspiration. Lancet 1970;1:1367–9.

28. Lin YJ, Yu YH. Reexpansion pulmonary edema after large-volume thoracentesis. Ann Thorac Surg 2011; 92:1550–1.

29. Mahfood S, Hix WR, Aaron BL, et al. Reexpansion pulmonary edema. Ann Thorac Surg 1988;45:340–5.

30. Feller-Kopman D, Berkowitz D, Boiselle P, et al. Large-volume thoracentesis and the risk of reexpansion pulmonary edema. Ann Thorac Surg 2007;84: 1656–61.

31. Jones PW, Moyers JP, Rogers JT, et al. Ultrasound guided thoracentesis. Is it a safer method? Chest 2003;123:418–23.

32. Havelock T, Teoh R, Laws D, et al. Pleural procedures and thoracic ultrasound: British Thoracic Society pleural disease guideline 2010. Thorax 2010;65:ii61–76.

33. Light RW, Jenkinson SG, Minh VD, et al. Observations on pleural fluid pressures as fluid is withdrawn during thoracentesis. Am Rev Respir Dis 1980;121: 799–804.

34. Huggins JT, Doelken P. Pleural manometry. Clin Chest Med 2006;27:229–40.

35. Feller-Kopman D, Walkey A, Berkowitz D, et al. The relationship of pleural pressure to symptoms development during therapeutic thoracentesis. Chest 2006;129:1556–60.

36. Gray H, Standring S, Ellis H, et al. Gray's anatomy: the anatomical basis of clinical practice. 39th edition. Edinburgh (United Kingdom): Elsevier Churchill Livingstone; 2005.

37. Rendina EA, Ciccone AM. The intercostal space. Thorac Surg Clin 2007;17:491–501.

38. Yoneyama H, Arahata M, Temaru R, et al. Evaluation of the risk of intercostal artery laceration during thoracentesis in elderly patients by using 3D-CT angiography. Intern Med 2010;49:289–92.

39. Rocha RP, Vengher A, Blanco A, et al. Size of the collateral intercostal artery in adults: anatomical considerations in relation to thoracentesis and thoracoscopy. Surg Radiol Anat 2002;24:23–6.

40. Salamonsen M, Ellis S, Paul E, et al. Thoracic ultrasound demonstrates variable location of the intercostal artery. Respiration 2012;83:323–9.

41. Choi S, Trieu J, Ridley L. Radiological review of intercostal artery: anatomical considerations when performing procedures via intercostal space. J Med Imaging Radiat Oncol 2010;54:302–6.

42. Peterson WG, Zimmerman R. Limited utility of chest radiograph after thoracentesis. Chest 2000;117: 1038–42.

43. Conner BD, Lee YC, Branca P, et al. Variations in pleural fluid WBC count and differential counts with different sample containers and different methods. Chest 2003;123:418–23.

44. Cheng DS, Rodriguez RM, Rogers J, et al. Comparison of pleural fluid pH values obtained using blood gas machine, pH meter, and pH indicator strip. Chest 1998;114:1368–72.

45. Goldstein LS, McCarthy K, Mehta AC, et al. Is direct collection of pleural fluid into a heparinized syringe important for determination of pleural pH? Chest 1997;112:707–8.

46. Rahman NM, Mishra EK, Davies HE, et al. Clinically important factors influencing the diagnostic measurement of pleural fluid pH and glucose. Am J Respir Crit Care Med 2008;178:483–90.

47. Sarodia BD, Goldstein LS, Laskowski DM, et al. Does pleural fluid pH change significantly at room temperature during the first hour following thoracentesis. Chest 2000;117:1043–8.

48. Spriggs AI, Boddington MM. The cytology of effusions. 2nd edition. New York: Grune & Stratton; 1968.

49. Naylor B, Schmidt RQ. The case for exfoliative cytology of serous effusions. Lancet 1964;1:711–2.

50. Naylor B. Pleural, peritoneal, and pericardial fluids. In: Bibbo M, editor. Comprehensive cytopathology. 2nd edition. Philadelphia: WB Sauders; 1997. p. 551–621.

51. Dekker A, Bupp PA. Cytology of serous effusions. An investigation into the usefulness of cell blocks versus smears. Am J Clin Pathol 1978;70:855–60.

52. Melamed MR. The cytological presentation of malignant lymphomas and related diseases in effusions. Cancer 1963;16:413–31.

53. Sallach SM, Sallach JA, Vasquez E, et al. Volume of pleural fluid required for diagnosis of pleural malignancy. Chest 2002;122:1913.

54. Abouzgheib W, Bartter T, Dagher H, et al. A prospective study of the volume of pleural fluid required for accurate diagnosis of malignant pleural effusion. Chest 2009;135:999.

55. Swiderek J, Morcos S, Donthireddy V, et al. Prospective study to determine the volume of pleural fluid required to diagnose malignancy. Chest 2010;137:68.

56. Capizzi SA, Prakash UB. Chest roentgenography after outpatient thoracentesis. Mayo Clin Proc 1998;73:948–50.

57. Doyle JJ, Hnatiuk OW, Torrington KG, et al. Necessity of routine chest roentgenography after thoracentesis. Ann Intern Med 1996;124:816–20.

58. Aleman C, Alegre J, Armadans L, et al. The value of chest roentgenography after thoracentesis. Am J Med 1999;107:340–3.

59. Moore C, Copel J. Point of care ultrasonography. N Engl J Med 2011;364:749–57.

60. Beckh S, Bolcskei PL, Lessnau KD. Real-time chest ultrasonography: a comprehensive review for the pulmonologist. Chest 2002;122:1759–73.

61. Kalokairinou-Motogna M, Maratou K, Paianid I, et al. Application of color Doppler ultrasound in the study of small pleural effusion. Med Ultrason 2010;12:12.

62. Duncan DR, Morgenthaler TI, Ryu JH, et al. Reducing iatrogenic risk in thoracentesis: establishing best practice via experiential training in a zero-risk environment. Chest 2009;135:1315–20.

63. Brooks A, Davies B, Smethhurst M, et al. Prospective evaluation of non-radiologist performed emergency abdominal ultrasound for haemoperitoneum. Emerg Med J 2004;21:e5.

64. Chalumeau-Lemoine L, Baudel JL, Das V, et al. Results of short-term training of naïve physicians in focused general ultrasonography in an intensive-care unit. Intensive Care Med 2009;35:1767–71.

65. ACGME program requirements for fellowship education in 2 pulmonary disease and critical care medicine (internal medicine), IV.A.5.a). (4). (m), Available at: www.acgme.org/acwebsite/rrc_140/140_prIndex.asp.

66. Kohan JM, Poe RH, Israel RH, et al. Value of chest ultrasonography versus decubitus roentgenography for thoracentesis. Am Rev Respir Dis 1986;133:1124–6.

67. Rao S, van Holsbeeck L, Musial JL, et al. A pilot study of comprehensive ultrasound education at the Wayne State University School of Medicine: a pioneer year review. J Ultrasound Med 2008;27:745–9.

68. Mathis G. Thoraxsonography-part I: chest wall and pleura. Praxis 2004;93:615–21.

69. Mayo P, Beaulieu Y, Doelken P, et al. American College of Chest Physicians/La Socié té de Ré animation de Langue Francaise statement on competence in critical care ultrasonography. Chest 2009;135:1050–60.

70. Kocijancic I, Vidmar K, Ivanovi-Herceg Z. Chest sonography versus lateral decubitus radiography in the diagnosis of small pleural effusions. J Clin Ultrasound 2003;31:69–74.

71. Diacon AH, Brutsche MH, Soler M. Accuracy of pleural puncture sites. A prospective comparison of clinical examination with ultrasound. Chest 2003;123:436–44.

72. Raptopoulos V, Davis LM, Lee G. Factors affecting the development of pneumothorax associated with thoracentesis. AJR Am J Roentgenol 1991;156:917–20.

73. Chen CH, Chen W, Chen HJ, et al. Transthoracic ultrasonography in predicting the outcome of small-bore catheter drainage in empyemas or complicated para-pneumonic effusions. Ultrasound Med Biol 2009;35:1468–74.

74. Medford AR, Agarawal S, Bennett JA, et al. Thoracic ultrasound prior to medical thoracoscopy improves pleural access and predicts fibrous septation. Respirology 2010;15:804–8.

75. Rantanen NW. Diseases of the thorax. Vet Clin North Am Equine Pract 1986;2:49–66.

76. Soldati G, Testa A, Sher S, et al. Occult traumatic pneumothorax: diagnostic accuracy of lung ultrasonography in the emergency department. Chest 2008;133:204–11.

77. Alrajhi K, Woo MY, Vaillancourt C. Test characteristics of ultrasonography for the detection of pneumothorax. A systematic review and meta-analysis. Chest 2012;141:703–8.

78. Rowan KR, Kirkpatrick AW, Liu D, et al. Traumatic pneumothorax detection with thoracic US: correlation with chest radiography and CT-Initial experience. Radiology 2002;225:210–4.

79. Galbois A, Ait-Oufella H, Baudel JL, et al. Pleural ultrasound compared with chest radiographic detection of pneumothorax resolution after drainage. Chest 2010;138:648–55.

80. Lichtenstein DA, Meziere G, Lascols N, et al. Ultrasound diagnosis of occult pneumothorax. Crit Care Med 2005;33:1231–8.

81. Lichenstein DA, Meziere G, Biderman P, et al. The comet-tail artifact: an interstitial sign of alveolar-interstitial syndrome. Am J Respir Crit Care Med 1997;156:1640–6.

82. Lichenstein D, Meziere G, Biderman P, et al. The "lung point": an ultrasound sign specific to pneumothorax. Intensive Care Med 2000;26:1434–40.

83. Lichenstein DA, Lascols N, Prin S, et al. The "lung pulse": an early ultrasound sign of complete atelectasis. Intensive Care Med 2003;29:2187–92.

84. Lichenstein DA, Meziere G. Relevance of lung ultrasound in the diagnosis of acute respiratory failure the BLUE protocol. Chest 2008;134:117–25.

85. Lichenstein DA, Meziere G, Biderman P, et al. The comet-tail artifact: an ultrasound sign ruling out pneumothorax. Intensive Care Med 1999;25:383–8.

86. Hooper C, Lee YC, Maskell N. Setting up a specialist pleural disease service. Respirology 2010;15:1028–36.

87. Mishra E, Davies HE, Lee Y. Malignant pleural disease in primary lung cancer. In: Spiro SG, Janes SM, Huber RM, editors. Thoracic malignancies. 3rd edition. Sheffield (United Kingdom): European Respirartory Society Journals Ltd; 2009. p. 138–335.

88. Brims FJ, Lansley SM, Waterer GW, et al. Empyema thoracis: new insights into an old disease. Eur Respir Rev 2010;19:220–8.

89. Roxburgh CS, Youngson CG, Townend JA, et al. Trends in pneumonia and empyema in Scottish children in the past 25 years. Arch Dis Child 2007;93:316–8.

90. Finley C, Clifton J, Fitzgerald JM, et al. Empyema: an increasing concern in Canada. Can Respir J 2008;15:85–9.

91. Farjah F, Symons RG, Krisnadasan B, et al. Management of pleural space infections: a population-based analysis. J Thorac Cardiovasc Surg 2007;133:346–51.

92. Heffner JE, Holgate ST, Chung KF, et al. The road ahead to respiratory health- experts chart future research directions. Respirology 2009;14:625–36.

The Evaluation and Clinical Application of Pleural Physiology

Jason Akulian, MD, MPH, Lonny Yarmus, DO,
David Feller-Kopman, MD*

KEYWORDS

• Pleura • Manometry • Lung entrapment • Trapped lung • Thoracentesis

KEY POINTS

• As the incidence of pleural disease continues to rise, the evaluation and clinical application of pleural physiology has become increasingly recognized in importance.
• Both pleural ultrasonography and manometry enhance understanding of underlying pleural pathology and physiology.
• Thoracic ultrasound should be used to guide all pleural procedures.
• Although further research is required to define the role of pleural manometry, measurement of Ppl is easily performed at the bedside, can help differentiate lung entrapment and trapped lung, allows for the safe removal of large effusions, and is a useful tool to aid in the selection of appropriate patients with malignant pleural effusions for pleurodesis.
• The application of real-time pathophysiologic data has enhanced our clinical decision making and continues to improve patient care.

Pleural disease affects approximately 1.5 million patients per year in the United States and remains one of the most commonly encountered entities by the chest physician.[1,2] The approach to evaluating pleural effusions has historically involved thoracentesis and pleural fluid analysis; however, full evaluation of lung, pleura, and chest wall pathophysiology via improvements in minimally invasive procedures, imaging, and pleural manometry has allowed for recent advances in the diagnosis and treatment of pleural disease.

Although investigations into pleural physiology through the measurement of intrapleural pressures have been undertaken for more than 120 years,[3] the clinical use of pleural manometry and its bedside applications have only recently been integrated into routine clinical practice. Additionally, the use of point-of-care ultrasound to assess the pleural space has increased tremendously. The use of bedside ultrasonography in the evaluation of the pleural space and lung parenchyma has been shown to be easily learned and applied, significantly affecting patient care and medical education.[4–6] The clinical application of pleural manometry gained favor in the early twentieth century, when the measurement of pleural pressure was used to confirm entry into the pleural space when inducing a pneumothorax for the treatment of tuberculosis. It was noted that some patients developed "unexpandable lung" due to parenchymal or visceral pleural scarring, with the

Conflicts of Interest/Disclosures: None.
Division of Pulmonary and Critical Care Medicine, The Johns Hopkins University School of Medicine, 1800 Orleans Street, Suite 7-125, Baltimore, MD 21287, USA
* Corresponding author.
E-mail address: dfellerk@jhmi.edu

formation of a pleural effusion ex vacuo.[7] The assessment of pleural pressure has more recently been used to help minimize the pressure-related complications known to occur during and after thoracentesis, as well as guide pleural palliation in patients with malignant effusions.[8,9] This review is written with the goal of improving the understanding of pleural physiology, and the pathophysiologic processes of unexpandable lung (ie, trapped lung and lung entrapment).

THE ANATOMY OF THE PLEURAL SPACE

The pleura is a thin, 5-layer membrane consisting of an outer fibroelastic layer, a subpleural highly vascularized loose connective tissue layer, a superficial elastic tissue layer, a submesothelial loose connective tissue layer, and a layer of mesothelium. During embryogenesis, the pleural space arises as a mesodermal cavity into and up-against which the developing lungs press and are eventually enveloped. The pleura directly adjacent to the lungs becomes the visceral pleura, then reflects at the hilum and becomes the parietal pleural when it comes in contact with the chest wall, mediastinum, and diaphragm. Once fully developed, the pleural space typically contains 0.5 to 2.0 mL of pleural fluid, allowing for close apposition of the visceral and parietal pleural. The multipotent mesothelial layer found on the inner lining of the pleural space is highly metabolically active, involves both cellular and humoral immunity, and plays an active role in pleural fluid production and reabsorption.[10,11]

PLEURAL PHYSIOLOGY
Pleural Fluid Formation

Pleural fluid originates from pleural capillaries via microvascular filtration across the pleural capillary endothelium and interstitium in series. The capillary endothelium accounts for most of the resistance to flow; however, the resistive properties of the endothelium and interstitium are additive. This point becomes significant when disease changes these resistances, resulting in the development of increased pleural fluid production. The formation and regulation of pleural fluid is driven by Starling forces (the gradient of hydrostatic and oncotic pressures found between the pleural space and opposing pleural capillary beds), solute flux, hydraulic conductivity (the resistive properties of the 2 membranes), total surface area, the solute reflection coefficient (the ability to restrict larger molecules), and the diffusive permeability of the pleural capillary endothelium and interstitium.[12]

These elements are expressed in the Starling equation:

Parietal Pleura:
$$Qf_{(parietal)} = Lp * A [(Pcap - Ppl) - \sigma d(\pi cap - \pi pl)]$$

Visceral Pleura:
$$Qf_{(visceral)} = Lp * A [(Pcap - Ppl) - \sigma d(\pi cap - \pi pl)]$$

Net Pleural Fluid Movement:
$$Qf_{(Total)} = Qf_{(parietal)} + Qf_{(visceral)}$$

Qf describes the liquid movement across the membrane, Lp is the filtration coefficient (water conductivity of the membrane), A is the surface area, P is the hydrostatic pressure of the capillary (Pcap) or pleura (Ppl), π is the oncotic pressure of the capillaries and pleural space, and σd is the solute reflection coefficient. The Starling equation should be calculated for both pleural surfaces to determine the net pleural fluid formation.

Extrapolating from animal models, the normal rate of pleural fluid production is believed to be approximately 0.01 mL/kg/h, and primarily arises from capillaries on the parietal pleura.[13] Likewise, pleural fluid is reabsorbed via stomata found on the caudal portions of the parietal pleura, which drain into lymphatics and have the ability to absorb fluid at a rate of approximately 0.28 mL/kg/h. Thus, for fluid to accumulate in the pleural space, 1 of 3 things must occur: the disease process must overwhelm the ability of the lymphatics to reabsorb fluid by substantially increasing pleural fluid production (28-fold), it must reduce the ability of the lymphatics to clear the fluid, or it must both increase production and decrease lymphatic clearance.

Pleural Pressure

Normal pleural pressure (Ppl) is slightly subatmospheric, approximately –3 to –5 cm H_2O, at functional residual capacity (FRC).[14] This is the result of the balance achieved by the elastic recoil forces of the lung exerting a force inward with the tendency of the chest wall to expand outward. Additionally, the pleural fluid itself contributes to the pressure in the pleural space. Under normal conditions, this total liquid volume is exceedingly small but does exert a small positive pressure on the total pleural pressure measured. Although pleural pressure is often referred to as a single pressure, it is actually the summation of multiple pressures occurring simultaneously: the pressure of pleural fluid, regional pleural surface deformation, and the weight of the lung in dependent areas of the thorax. These forces result in a pleural liquid pressure that is slightly more subatmospheric than one would expect based solely on the recoil pressures of the lung and chest wall.[15]

Several theories have been proposed to explain regional differences in pleural pressure as effusions accumulate.[12,15–18] These theories account for the hydrostatic gradients that result from a column of fluid in the chest, as well as changes in deformation forces as the lung and chest wall become separated by the effusion.[12,16,18] As fluid accumulates in the pleural space, the forces of deformation are in part released, and 3 distinct pressure zones are created. In the upper zone, the thickness of the pleural fluid is normal and the pleural liquid pressure remains lower than the pleural surface pressure. In the middle zone, as pleural liquid thickness and starts to increase, pleural liquid pressure becomes zero and pleural liquid pressure equalizes with pleural surface pressure. In the lower zone, the pleural liquid pressure becomes positive and the lung and chest wall are pushed apart.[14,19] This concept represents the hydrostatic theory of pleural pressure that pleural liquid is in hydrostatic equilibrium maintained by a vertical gradient in pleural pressure of 1 cm H_2O/cm height.[20]

Another model of pleural forces maintains that pleural liquid pressure is always equal to pleural surface pressure. This concept suggests that pressure gradients owing to gravity and regional differences in pleural surface pressure drive a small viscous flow of fluid in the pleural space, thereby leading to the presence of a small, continuous layer of pleural fluid throughout the thorax and no direct contact between the lung and chest wall (ie, the visceral and parietal pleural surfaces do not come into contact).[21] As pleural fluid accumulates, the viscous resistance to flow falls rapidly and the gradient in the pleural pressure approaches that of the hydrostatic pressure gradient equal to 1 cm H_2O/cm of height of the effusion.[15,16,21]

Measurement of pleural liquid and surface pressure in the normal pleural space is technically challenging because the normal pleural space is only approximately 20 μm in thickness, and the insertion of any device into the pleural space will create deformation forces not present before the insertion of the device.[12] Although there continues to be great debate between the 2 dominant theories of normal pleural pressure physiology,[12,22] the concepts at the center of this debate are likely only of practical importance at the termination of a thoracentesis, when a physiologic amount (5–8 mL) of pleural fluid remains. In the presence of even a small effusion (less than 500 mL), one can measure Ppl with a variety of techniques as the viscous resistance to flow becomes negligible. The pressure measured, therefore, is an accurate representation of the hydrostatic pressure in the effusion at the level of the catheter/transducer.

There has been some suggestion that when measuring Ppl, the height of the manometer relative to the effusion is insignificant.[23] This was hypothesized by applying Pascal's law, which states that in an enclosed system such as the chest, pressure is transmitted equally in all directions, and will exert the same force equally on the lung, chest wall, and manometer regardless of where the needle is inserted. This is in contrast to an open system, where the only force is that of gravity.[15] When applying these theories in a clinical setting, such as a pleural effusion, one must take into account that a hydrostatic pressure gradient of 1 cm H_2O/cm height *is present*, and so the pressure read by the manometer represents Ppl at a specific level, not the pressure throughout the hydrothorax. With the removal of pleural fluid and a reduction in the height of the fluid column above the catheter, the influence of the hydrostatic pressure gradient lessens. The measured Ppl, therefore, *does not* depend on the location of the catheter tip within the effusion; rather, it depends on the zero reference level; ie, the level at which the measuring system would register zero pressure if opened to atmosphere. The operator should place the catheter in a site in which a moderate amount of fluid is present to minimize risk of injuring the lung or intra-abdominal organs. Thereafter, he or she should direct the catheter to the most dependent part of the effusion. This has the potential benefits of maximizing the amount of fluid that is able to be removed while minimizing the risk of complications and creating deformation forces from the contact of the catheter with the lung. By establishing the zero reference level for the system near the top of the effusion, one will get a better estimate of the pressure in the pleural space that is a consequence primarily of the forces exerted by the lung and chest with less confounding of measurements caused by the hydrostatic fluid column above the transducer. With the catheter entry site in a more dependent position, the initial influence of the hydrostatic fluid column will be larger than at the terminal part of the thoracentesis when there is less fluid above the catheter.

PLEURAL ULTRASONOGRAPHY

The use of ultrasonography has been increasing among pulmonary and critical care physicians to aid in the diagnosis and management of patients with pleural effusion. Ultrasound can be used to identify even small effusions, and has been shown to improve the yield and reduce the risk of therapeutic thoracentesis and chest tube placement.[24,25] Please refer to the article by Sachdeva and colleagues elsewhere in this issue for further descriptions of this procedure. For completeness, ultrasound is discussed briefly here.

The presence of pleural fluid provides an excellent acoustic window that allows examination of the parietal and visceral pleura, as well as the pleural effusion itself. Examination of the pleural space is best performed with a 3.5-MHz to 5.0-MHz transducer, which provides both sufficient penetration and resolution.[26] Compared with the isoechoic reference of the liver or spleen, pleural fluid is usually hypoechoic (darker), and the air-filled lung is hyperechoic (brighter) (**Fig. 1**). With inspiration, the lung becomes more hyperechoic, and a dynamic, respirophasic "sliding" or "gliding" movement of the lung is seen, confirming that the hypoechoic area is fluid as opposed to tissue.[27] Although hypoechoic fluid can be either transudative or exudative, hyperechoic fluid is generally exudative.[28,29]

Although physical examination findings or a recent chest x-ray or computed tomography (CT) scan can all be used to help diagnose the presence and location of fluid,[25] ultrasound is clearly more sensitive for detecting pleural effusions than a lateral decubitus chest radiograph, and is also better able to predict the nature of the fluid.[30-32] When compared with CT scanning as the gold standard, ultrasonography of the chest has been found to have a 95% sensitivity for detecting pleural lesions in patients with a "white out" on chest radiograph.[33] Another clear benefit is the portability of the ultrasound machine, which is easily brought to the bedside, as opposed to transporting patients to the CT scanner. The time required to perform an ultrasound examination to evaluate for the presence of an effusion is quite small, averaging only approximately 2 minutes.[34]

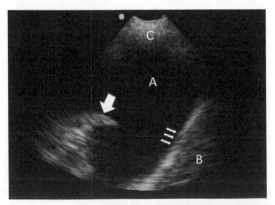

Fig. 1. Thoracic ultrasound of a pleural effusion. *Large arrow* shows hyperechoic lung; *small arrows* show diaphragm. (A) Large hypoechoic pleural effusion. (B) Hyperechoic liver. (C) Chest wall.

Guidance for Thoracentesis and Tube Thoracostomy

Generally considered to be a safe procedure, thoracentesis carries with it the risk of pneumothorax, injury to adjacent organs, and procedure failure. Several studies have shown the use of ultrasound during thoracentesis to be associated with a significant reduction in the rate of pneumothorax, even in patients receiving mechanical ventilation.[4,24,35-41]

Perhaps as important in reducing complications, ultrasonography has also been shown to reduce "near-misses" caused by inaccurate selection of the procedure site. In the study by Kohan and colleagues,[42] 58% of clinically attempted "dry taps" were found to be subdiaphragmatic. Diacon and colleagues[43] found that ultrasonography decreased the number of potentially dangerous needle-insertion sites and increased the rate of accurate site selection when compared with physical examination and chest radiograph localization.

The use of ultrasound to guide pleural access should be performed just before the procedure. When used as an "X marks the spot" technique with the ultrasound being performed in one location of the hospital followed by transfer of the patient to another location for the procedure, no difference in rates of complication were noted when compared with procedures in which the site was chosen clinically.[37,42] These findings have led the British Thoracic Society to conclude that thoracic ultrasound should be used for all pleural procedures and that marking of the procedure site using ultrasonography remotely from where the procedure is to be performed should not be attempted.[25]

PLEURAL MANOMETRY

Clinical application of pleural physiology begins with the measurement of intrapleural pressures. Pleural pressure can be measured with several techniques, including a U-shaped water manometer,[19] an "overdamped" water manometer,[21] or sophisticated electronic transducer systems that allow sampling frequencies of several hertz and provide the ability to store data for further analysis. A benefit of the U-shaped manometer is that it is relatively inexpensive and is easily performed by using the syringe-pump system available with most thoracentesis kits. A disadvantage, however, is that it may be difficult to accurately record values because of the pleural pressure swings associated with inspiration and expiration. Doelken and colleagues[21] recently described their use of an overdamped water manometer that uses a 22-gauge needle as a resistor, and has shown excellent correlation to the electronic system ($r = 0.97$). The benefits of this system are that it is relatively easy to set up, and it provides real-time *mean* Ppl without the large respiratory-related swings that are encountered with systems that are not damped. Electronic transducer systems can be configured for standard intensive care unit (ICU) monitors. Because these monitors are not calibrated to measure negative pressure, however, one needs to calibrate an "offset" or an adjustment in the actual height of the transducer relative to the zero reference level such that negative numbers can be recorded. Additionally, ICU hemodynamic transducers report data in mm Hg, as compared with the standard cm H_2O typically used for Ppl measurements. This problem is easily resolved by using the conversion factor of 1 mm Hg = 1.36 cm H_2O. A clear advantage of using an electronic transducer system is that it provides the capability to review the Ppl curves after the data have been collected, and thereby enables analysis of pressure anywhere in the respiratory cycle (ie, at end inspiration and end expiration), as well as the opportunity to calculate mean Ppl. Most experts currently report mean or end-expiratory (ie, at FRC) Ppl. It may be, however, that end inspiratory pressure is most relevant as a possible risk factor for the development of pressure-related complications, such as re-expansion pulmonary edema.

Assessing Pleural Elastance

Although controversy regarding the utility of pleural manometry exists, there is agreement that the technique is useful in guiding clinical decision making in the setting of malignant pleural effusion.[44,45] Accurate assessment of Ppl at the time of the insertion of the catheter and periodically while fluid is being removed can provide information to assist in the diagnosis of the effusion and the presence of unexpandable lung. In 1980, Light and colleagues[19] used a water-filled U-shaped manometer connected to an Abram needle with the goal of determining the clinical utility of pleural manometry, and to evaluate the safety of large-volume thoracentesis. Pleural fluid was removed until the Ppl fell to less than –20 cm H_2O, no more fluid could be obtained, or until patients developed symptoms described as more than minimal in severity. Although the initial Ppl varied widely (–21 cm H_2O to +8 cm H_2O), an initial pressure of less than –5 cm H_2O was seen only in patients with malignant effusions or trapped lung. Light and colleagues[19] also measured pleural elastance (Eps, change in pressure in the pleural space divided by the volume of fluid removed measured

in liters) and described 3 distinct Eps curves: (1) removal of a large amount of fluid with minimal change in pressure (normal pleural elastance, as can be seen in patients with hepatic hydrothorax or congestive heart failure), (2) a relatively normal initial curve followed by a sharp drop in pressure (lung entrapment), and (3) a negative initial pressure with a rapid drop in pressure (trapped lung) (**Fig. 2**). An Eps greater than 25 cm H_2O/L was seen in patients with malignancy or trapped lung.

Since Light and colleagues'[19] study of Eps, assessment of Ppl through manometry has been shown to be predictive in identifying patients appropriate for pleurodesis. Lan and colleagues[9] found that none of the patients with an Eps greater than 19 cm H_2O (after draining 500 mL of fluid) had successful pleurodesis compared with 98% of those with an Eps less than 19 cm H_2O (after draining 500 mL of fluid) who achieved pleurodesis. Pleural pressure has also been shown to correlate with the development of chest discomfort during thoracentesis[8]; its measurement can aid in identification of the etiology of post-thoracentesis pneumothorax.[8,46]

For the practicing clinician it may seem daunting to choose a method and then to perform pleural manometry. A simple method used by the authors involves the use of the catheter insertion site as the zero point then measuring the distance, negative or positive, from this where spontaneous flow ceases from the syringe connecting tube, which

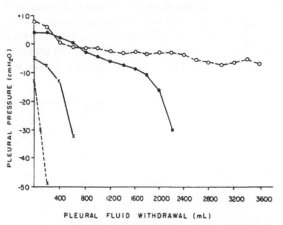

Fig. 2. Pleural elastance curves. *Unfilled circle* shows normal pleural elastance with minimal change in pressure. *Filled circle* shows lung entrapment, normal initial curve followed by a sharp drop in pressure. X-trapped lung, negative initial pressure with a rapid drop. (*Reprinted from* Light RW, Jenkinson SG, Minh VD, et al. Observations on pleural fluid pressures as fluid is withdrawn during thoracentesis. Am Rev Respir Dis 1980;121:799–804. Official Journal of the American Thoracic Society. Copyright © 2012 American Thoracic Society; with permission.)

acts as an ad hoc U-shaped manometer. Another method involves the use of commercially available handheld pressure transducers, currently being validated in comparative clinical studies. At this time, it is impossible to recommend one method of measuring Ppl over another, but we strongly suggest becoming familiar with a system that can be easily used and replicated on each patient at your local institution and manometry be performed on all thoracenteses (**Fig. 3**).

RE-EXPANSION PULMONARY EDEMA

During a thoracentesis, one would ideally like to remove as much fluid as is safely possible. The goals of completely draining the pleural space include maximizing symptomatic relief, sparing the patient multiple procedures, increasing the yield of other diagnostic tests, such as a post-thoracentesis CT scan, and documenting lung re-expansion before attempts at pleurodesis. Pleural manometry allows for the safe drainage of large volumes of fluid as well as avoiding the pressure-related consequences of thoracentesis, such as re-expansion pulmonary edema (RPE). Light and colleagues[19] originally showed that if thoracentesis was terminated when the Ppl dropped to -20 cm H_2O, RPE was avoided despite removing large quantities of fluid. They concluded that, "…as the operator cannot easily estimate pleural pressure…therapeutic thoracentesis should be limited to 1000 mL unless pleural pressures are monitored." A pressure of -20 cm H_2O was arbitrarily chosen based on prior animal studies investigating pneumothorax[47,48] showing a minimal risk of RPE if Ppl was kept above -20 mm Hg (approximately -27 cm H_2O), but a significant risk was present with Ppl of -40 mm Hg (approximately -54 cm H_2O). The above quote has led to most clinicians terminating thoracentesis after removing 1000 to 1500 mL without regard to the amount of remaining pleural fluid, the potential benefit of removing that fluid, or consideration of pleural pressure.

In a study of 61 patients, Villena and colleagues[49] used manometry to define the relationships of Ppl to the underlying diagnosis as well as complications of therapeutic thoracentesis. They reported no association between a negative initial Ppl and procedural complications; however, an initial Ppl less than -4 cm H_2O and an Eps greater than 33 cm H_2O/L was associated with unexpandable lung. There were no cases of RPE, despite a mean removal of 1.45 L of pleural fluid.

In addition, Feller-Kopman and colleagues[50] published the results from more than 185 large-volume (>1 L) thoracenteses (mean 1.67 L, range 1000 mL–6550 mL), with only 1 patient developing clinically significant RPE. Feller-Kopman and colleagues[50] showed no relationship in the development of RPE to the volume of pleural fluid removed, opening or closing Ppl, Eps, or symptoms during the thoracentesis, suggesting that RPE is a rare event (incidence of 0.54% in this study). As such, we recommend manometry be used on all pleural drainage procedures and recommend cessation of thoracentesis if Ppl is less than -20 cm H_2O or the patient develops chest discomfort.

THE UNEXPANDABLE LUNG: TRAPPED LUNG AND LUNG ENTRAPMENT

The unexpandable lung, historically referred to as "trapped lung," has long been recognized as the

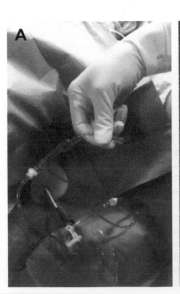
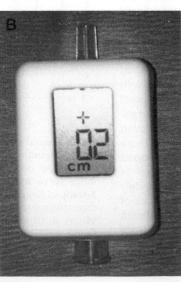

Fig. 3. (*A*) A convenient means of bedside pleural manometry and determining when spontaneous flow ceases. (*B*) A transducer being evaluated for commercial use.

sequelae of active or remote pleural and/or parenchymal disease (**Fig. 4**).[51] This has led to an attempt at characterization of the underlying pathophysiology through the use of the terms "lung entrapment" and "trapped lung." Although confusing terms, lung entrapment and trapped lung describe different time points in the pathophysiology of the unexpandable lung.

Lung entrapment describes lung parenchyma rendered unexpandable after thoracentesis by an active process, such as visceral pleural inflammation or malignancy, endobronchial obstruction, or diseases that increase the elastic recoil of the lung, such as interstitial lung disease or lymphangitic carcinomatosis. Patients often present with dyspnea related to the effusion as well as with signs and symptoms attributable to the underlying disease. Chest discomfort or other signs of pleural inflammation, such as fever, may also be present. Chest radiography may show a contralateral mediastinal shift. The effusion associated with lung entrapment is typically exudative, because of the active underlying inflammation or tumor. As the lung is not able to fully expand with drainage of the pleural fluid, although the initial pressure may be positive, Ppl drops steeply toward the terminal portion of the thoracentesis. The *mean* elastance can be low, although the terminal elastance calculated from removal of the last aliquot of fluid may be quite high.[51–53] With normal healing of the underlying process, the effusion may completely resolve without any resultant thickening of the visceral pleura.

Trapped lung, on the other hand, represents the sequelae of remote pleural inflammation resulting in visceral pleural scarring and/orthickening.[51] The result is a lung that behaves as if it is much stiffer (ie, has a reduced compliance), creating a highly negative Ppl during inspiration as the chest wall moves outward and the trapped lung remains essentially static, resisting expansion or deformation. Excessively negative Ppl compared with the normal state is present during both inhalation and exhalation and shifts the balance of Starling forces that are responsible for the production of pleural fluid, such that more fluid moves into the pleural space. The accumulation of fluid attributable to this process is described as "effusion ex-vacuo." Because there is no active pleural inflammation, patients typically present with a chronic, asymptomatic effusion that is identified on routine physical examination or chest radiograph. As the pleural fluid formation results from an excess of negative pleural pressure, it is rare to see contralateral mediastinal shift on a chest radiograph, even in the presence of a moderate to large effusion. Similarly, because the effusion is attributable to an imbalance of hydrostatic forces, it is almost always transudative in nature. Given that most of these patients are asymptomatic, therapy aimed at the pleural effusion is usually not required. Should the patient have exertional dyspnea resulting from a restrictive ventilatory defect because of the pleural scarring, decortication will likely be required to expand the underlying lung.

As described previously, lung entrapment and trapped lung are part of a continuum of the underlying disease, and as such, one may occasionally obtain pleural fluid results that fall in the exudative range, even in the setting of trapped lung physiology, depending on when the thoracentesis is performed in the healing process.[52] Pleural manometry remains the method of choice for detecting unexpandable lung.[51]

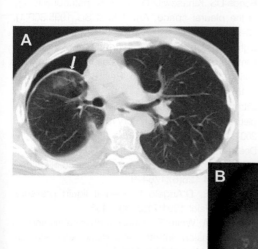

Fig. 4. (*A*) Chest CT scan showing visceral pleural thickening (*arrow*), nonexpandable lung and pneumothorax after thoracoscopy, pleural biopsy, and thoracentesis. (*B*) Visceral pleural thickening/peel seen during thoracoscopy.

In an attempt to define the etiology of unexpandable lung, Huggins and colleagues[52] described the use of "air-contrast" CT scan to visualize visceral pleural thickness in 247 consecutive patients undergoing pleural manometry during thoracentesis. They identified 11 patients with a clinical diagnosis of trapped lung. All of these patients developed a mean Ppl of less than −25 cm H_2O and had prior pleural fluid analysis that was not suggestive of malignancy or pleural inflammation. At the termination of the therapeutic thoracentesis, they instilled atmospheric air, a "diagnostic pneumothorax," with the goal of raising the Ppl to a more physiologic mean of −5 cm H_2O and alleviating the patient's chest discomfort associated with the drop in Ppl. The air-contrast CT scan confirmed visceral pleural thickening in all 11 patients. As expected, all of these patients had a high pleural elastance (Eps >19 cm H_2O/L). Based on their findings, they recommend using the air-contrast CT as part of the diagnostic approach to patients with trapped lung as a way to minimize additional pleural interventions, such as attempts at pleurodesis, which will have a low likelihood of success.

SUMMARY

As the incidence of pleural disease continues to rise, the evaluation and clinical application of pleural physiology has become increasingly recognized in importance. Both pleural ultrasonography and manometry enhance understanding of underlying pleural pathology and physiology. Thoracic ultrasound should be to guide all pleural procedures. Although further research is required to define the role of pleural manometry, measurement of Ppl is easily performed at the bedside, can help differentiate lung entrapment and trapped lung, allows for the safe removal of large effusions, and is a useful tool to aid in the selection of appropriate patients with malignant pleural effusions for pleurodesis. The application of real-time pathophysiologic data has enhanced our clinical decision making and continues to improve patient care.

REFERENCES

1. Light RW. Pleural diseases. 4th edition. Philadelphia: Lippincott Williams & Wilkins; 2001.
2. Maskell N. British thoracic society pleural disease guidelines—2010 update. Thorax 2010;65(8):667–9.
3. Quincke H. Ueber den Druck in Transudaten. Dtsch Arch Klin Med 1878;21:453–68.
4. Mayo PH, Goltz HR, Tafreshi M, et al. Safety of ultrasound-guided thoracentesis in patients receiving mechanical ventilation. Chest 2004;125(3):1059–62.
5. Feller-Kopman D. Ultrasound-guided thoracentesis. Chest 2006;129(6):1709–14.
6. Rozycki GS, Pennington SD, Feliciano DV. Surgeon-performed ultrasound in the critical care setting: its use as an extension of the physical examination to detect pleural effusion. J Trauma 2001;50(4):636–42.
7. Farber J, Lincoln NS. The unexpandable lung. Am Rev Tuberc 1939;40:704–9.
8. Feller-Kopman D, Walkey A, Berkowitz D, et al. The relationship of pleural pressure to symptom development during therapeutic thoracentesis. Chest 2006;129(6):1556–60.
9. Lan RS, Lo SK, Chuang ML, et al. Elastance of the pleural space: a predictor for the outcome of pleurodesis in patients with malignant pleural effusion. Ann Intern Med 1997;126(10):768–74.
10. Wang NS. Anatomy of the pleura. Clin Chest Med 1998;19(2):229–40.
11. Jantz MA, Antony VB. Pathophysiology of the pleura. Respiration 2008;75(2):121–33.
12. Lai-Fook SJ. Pleural mechanics and fluid exchange. Physiol Rev 2004;84(2):385–410.
13. Antunes G, Neville E, Duffy J, et al. BTS guidelines for the management of malignant pleural effusions. Thorax 2003;58(Suppl 2):ii29–38. PMCID: 1766015.
14. Broaddus V, Light R. Disorders of the pleura: general principles and diagnostic approach. In: Murray J, Nadel J, editors. Textbook of respiratory medicine. Philadelphia: W.B. Saunders Company; 1994. p. 2145–63.
15. Agostoni E. Mechanics of the pleural space. Physiol Rev 1972;52(1):57–128.
16. Lai-Fook SJ. Mechanics of the pleural space: fundamental concepts. Lung 1987;165(5):249–67.
17. Agostoni E, D'Angelo E. Thickness and pressure of the pleural liquid at various heights and with various hydrothoraces. Respir Physiol 1969;6(3):330–42.
18. Boggs DS, Kinasewitz GT. Review: pathophysiology of the pleural space. Am J Med Sci 1995;309(1):53–9.
19. Light RW, Jenkinson SG, Minh VD, et al. Observations on pleural fluid pressures as fluid is withdrawn during thoracentesis. Am Rev Respir Dis 1980;121(5):799–804.
20. Mitrouska I, Klimathianaki M, Siafakas NM. Effects of pleural effusion on respiratory function. Can Respir J 2004;11(7):499–503.
21. Doelken P, Huggins JT, Pastis NJ, et al. Pleural manometry: technique and clinical implications. Chest 2004;126(6):1764–9.
22. Agostoni E, D'Angelo E. Pleural liquid pressure. J Appl Physiol 1991;71(2):393–403.
23. Bernstein A, White FZ. Unusual physical findings in pleural effusion: intrathoracic manometric studies. Ann Intern Med 1952;37(4):733–8.
24. Gordon CE, Feller-Kopman D, Balk EM, et al. Pneumothorax following thoracentesis: a systematic

review and meta-analysis. Arch Intern Med 2010; 170(4):332–9.

25. Havelock T, Teoh R, Laws D, et al. Pleural procedures and thoracic ultrasound: British Thoracic Society Pleural Disease Guideline 2010. Thorax 2010;65(Suppl 2):ii61–76.

26. Beckh S, Bolcskei PL, Lessnau KD. Real-time chest ultrasonography: a comprehensive review for the pulmonologist. Chest 2002;122(5):1759–73.

27. Marks WM, Filly RA, Callen PW. Real-time evaluation of pleural lesions: new observations regarding the probability of obtaining free fluid. Radiology 1982; 142(1):163–4.

28. Yang PC, Luh KT, Chang DB, et al. Value of sonography in determining the nature of pleural effusion: analysis of 320 cases. AJR Am J Roentgenol 1992; 159(1):29–33.

29. Tu CY, Hsu WH, Hsia TC, et al. Pleural effusions in febrile medical ICU patients: chest ultrasound study. Chest 2004;126(4):1274–80.

30. Eibenberger KL, Dock WI, Ammann ME, et al. Quantification of pleural effusions: sonography versus radiography. Radiology 1994;191(3):681–4.

31. Vignon P, Chastagner C, Berkane V, et al. Quantitative assessment of pleural effusion in critically ill patients by means of ultrasonography. Crit Care Med 2005;33(8):1757–63.

32. Balik M, Plasil P, Waldauf P, et al. Ultrasound estimation of volume of pleural fluid in mechanically ventilated patients. Intensive Care Med 2006;32(2):318–21.

33. Yu CJ, Yang PC, Wu HD, et al. Ultrasound study in unilateral hemithorax opacification. Image comparison with computed tomography. Am Rev Respir Dis 1993;147(2):430–4.

34. Tayal VS, Nicks BA, Norton HJ. Emergency ultrasound evaluation of symptomatic nontraumatic pleural effusions. Am J Emerg Med 2006;24(7):782–6.

35. Grogan DR, Irwin RS, Channick R, et al. Complications associated with thoracentesis. A prospective, randomized study comparing three different methods. Arch Intern Med 1990;150(4):873–7.

36. Jones PW, Moyers JP, Rogers JT, et al. Ultrasound-guided thoracentesis: is it a safer method? Chest 2003;123(2):418–23.

37. Raptopoulos V, Davis LM, Lee G, et al. Factors affecting the development of pneumothorax associated with thoracentesis. AJR Am J Roentgenol 1991; 156(5):917–20.

38. Barnes TW, Morgenthaler TI, Olson EJ, et al. Sonographically guided thoracentesis and rate of pneumothorax. J Clin Ultrasound 2005;33(9):442–6.

39. Hirsch JH, Rogers JV, Mack LA. Real-time sonography of pleural opacities. AJR Am J Roentgenol 1981;136(2):297–301.

40. Weingardt JP, Guico RR, Nemcek AA Jr, et al. Ultrasound findings following failed, clinically directed thoracenteses. J Clin Ultrasound 1994; 22(7):419–26.

41. Lichtenstein D, Hulot JS, Rabiller A, et al. Feasibility and safety of ultrasound-aided thoracentesis in mechanically ventilated patients. Intensive Care Med 1999; 25(9):955–8.

42. Kohan JM, Poe RH, Israel RH, et al. Value of chest ultrasonography versus decubitus roentgenography for thoracentesis. Am Rev Respir Dis 1986;133(6): 1124–6.

43. Diacon AH, Brutsche MH, Soler M. Accuracy of pleural puncture sites: a prospective comparison of clinical examination with ultrasound. Chest 2003; 123(2):436–41.

44. Feller-Kopman D. Point: should pleural manometry be performed routinely during thoracentesis? Yes. Chest 2012;141(4):844–5.

45. Maldonado F, Mullon JJ. Counterpoint: should pleural manometry be performed routinely during thoracentesis? No. Chest 2012;141(4):846–8 [discussion: 8–9].

46. Heidecker J, Huggins JT, Sahn SA, et al. Pathophysiology of pneumothorax following ultrasound-guided thoracentesis. Chest 2006;130(4):1173–84.

47. Pavlin J, Cheney FW Jr. Unilateral pulmonary edema in rabbits after reexpansion of collapsed lung. J Appl Physiol 1979;46(1):31–5.

48. Miller WC, Toon R, Palat H, et al. Experimental pulmonary edema following re-expansion of pneumothorax. Am Rev Respir Dis 1973;108(3):654–6.

49. Villena V, Lopez-Encuentra A, Pozo F, et al. Measurement of pleural pressure during therapeutic thoracentesis. Am J Respir Crit Care Med 2000; 162(4 Pt 1):1534–8.

50. Feller-Kopman D, Berkowitz D, Boiselle P, et al. Large-volume thoracentesis and the risk of reexpansion pulmonary edema. Ann Thorac Surg 2007; 84(5):1656–61.

51. Huggins JT, Doelken P, Sahn SA. The unexpandable lung. F1000 Med Rep 2010;2:77. PMCID: 2981182.

52. Huggins JT, Sahn SA, Heidecker J, et al. Characteristics of trapped lung: pleural fluid analysis, manometry, and air-contrast chest CT. Chest 2007;131(1):206–13.

53. Feller-Kopman D, Parker MJ, Schwartzstein RM. Assessment of pleural pressure in the evaluation of pleural effusions. Chest 2009;135(1):201–9.

The Light Criteria
The Beginning and Why they are Useful 40 Years Later

Richard W. Light, MD

KEYWORDS

• Light criteria • Pleural effusion • Transudative effusion

KEY POINTS

- The Light criteria serve as a good starting point in the separation of transudates from exudates.
- The Light criteria misclassify about 25% of transudates as exudates, and most of these patients are on diuretics.
- If a patient is thought likely to have a disease that produces a transudative pleural effusion but the Light criteria suggest an exudate by only a small margin, the serum–pleural fluid protein gradient should be examined.
- If this is greater than 3.1 gm/dL, the patient in all probability has a transudative effusion.
- If the gradient is less than 3.1 gm/dL, either the NT-pro-BNP level in the pleural fluid or the serum–pleural fluid albumin gradient can be measured.
- Either an NT-pro-BNP greater than 1300 pg/mL or an albumin gradient greater than 1.2 gm/dL indicate that the effusion is a transudate.

It has been 40 years since I published the article[1] describing what came to be known as the Light criteria. I thought that it might be appropriate to begin this article by detailing how that article came about.

THE DEVELOPMENT OF THE LIGHT CRITERIA

When I was an intern in medicine at Johns Hopkins Hospital in Baltimore, Maryland, in 1968 to 1969, there was a period when a large percentage of my patients had a pleural effusion. The chief resident, Dr Richard Winterbauer, made rounds around midnight and always asked me what the thoracentesis revealed. At that time, we routinely measured the cell count and differential, glucose, and protein, and performed smears and cultures on the pleural fluid. I asked Dr Winterbauer the significance of the various pleural fluid findings

and, for the most part, neither he nor anybody else had a scientific answer.

It was at this time that additional measurements were first being made on blood, such as the lactic dehydrogenase (LDH), aspartate aminotransferase (AST), and alanine aminotransferase (ALT). At about the same time, blood gas machines became available that would allow the accurate measurement of pH, P_{CO_2}, and P_{O_2} of body fluids. I theorized that some of these new measurements might be useful in the differential diagnosis of pleural effusions. After doing a literature review, I developed 2 hypotheses. The first was that the pH of pleural fluid would be lower in tuberculous pleural effusions than in other exudative pleural effusions. The basis for this hypothesis was an article in the *Scandinavian Journal of Respiratory Disease* that purported to show this.[2] My second hypothesis was that LDH isoenzymes would be

Disclosures: The author has nothing to disclose related to this publication.
Division of Allergy/Pulmonary/Critical Care, Vanderbilt University Medical Center, Vanderbilt University, 1161 21st Avenue South, Nashville, TN 37232, USA
E-mail address: Rlight98@yahoo.com

useful in the differential diagnosis of exudative pleural effusions. To get the absolute value of the LDH isoenzymes, I needed to have the total LDH in the pleural fluid and the serum. A previous study on pleural fluid LDH concluded that the pleural fluid LDH was increased in malignant pleural effusions compared with other pleural effusions.[3] I submitted a proposal to the Institutional Review Board and received their approval. The blood gas machine was in the pulmonary function laboratory and I could measure all of the pleural fluid pH myself. The clinical laboratory measured the protein, LDH, and glucose in the serum and pleural fluid without charge. However, I did have to come up with some funds to pay for the LDH isoenzymes. I received a small grant from Johns Hopkins Hospital to fund this.

To get called when patients with pleural effusions were admitted, I made a deal with my fellow interns and residents. If they would call me when they did a thoracentesis, I would do the cell count and differential on the pleural fluid; duties for which they would normally be responsible. I quickly found out that, with this arrangement, I got called often in the middle of the night about pleural effusions.

One of the first patients I studied was a young man with an exudative lymphocytic effusion. His pleural fluid pH was 7.40. The patient turned out to have caseating granulomas on the needle biopsy of his pleura; so much for the first hypothesis. Soon thereafter, another patient had a pleural fluid pH of 6.95. The pleural fluid was clear yellow and the pleural fluid glucose was not reduced. However, the pleural fluid grew *Streptococcus pneumoniae* and the patient eventually developed a frank pneumococcal empyema. This case was the first to suggest that a low pleural fluid pH might be an indicator of a complicated parapneumonic effusion.[4]

I subsequently studied more than 150 pleural effusions in a 2-year period. I submitted an abstract of my preliminary findings to the American Thoracic Society for their annual meeting in 1971. The abstract was rejected. I was devastated.

In early 1971, when I was a pulmonary fellow, Johns Hopkins had a reunion for some of its alumni. My mentor, Dr Wilmot C. Ball, Jr, suggested that I present something on the pleural fluid that I had been studying. At that time, transudates and exudates were usually separated by using a protein level of 3.0 gm/dL.[5] I elected to see how this would work on my set of pleural effusions. On a rainy, sleety Sunday in Baltimore, Maryland, I spent several hours with a pencil and graph paper plotting protein levels, LDH levels, and ratios of protein and LDH in the serum and pleural fluid.

When I examined my plots, it was obvious that no single value of any of these measurements correctly identified all transudates and exudates. If the cutoff was made high enough that all transudates were below the cutoff level, then some exudates would be classified as transudates. My objective at that time was to identify all exudates correctly. Therefore I elected to make the cutoff points such that no transudates were above the line. I noticed that, when I did this, some exudates were in the transudative range for each of the measurements. However, I also noticed that, if I used 3 different cutoff levels such that no transudates were above the cutoff line, I could identify almost all transudates and exudates correctly. The 3 cutoff points that I found were a protein ratio greater than 0.5, an LDH ratio greater than 0.6, and an absolute pleural fluid LDH greater than two-thirds of the upper normal limit for serum. An exudative effusion met at least 1 of these 3 criteria, whereas a transudative effusion met none.

I presented these data to the alumni and they did not seem particularly impressed. I also submitted an abstract on the separation of transudates by the criteria listed earlier to the American College of Physicians in 1972.[6] It was accepted for an oral presentation in Atlantic City. This oral presentation was the only one that I ever participated in where the audience graded the contents of the presentation. I got, at most, average marks; certainly nothing to suggest that these cutoff levels would still be in use 40 years later. Nevertheless, I wrote the article and submitted it to the *Annals of Internal Medicine*. It was accepted with minimal revisions.[1]

There are several lessons to be learned from my experience in developing the Light criteria. First, if you want people to cooperate with you on your research, you need to make it worthwhile for them. In this case, I did some of the work that they would otherwise have to do. Second, although research is best done when it is hypothesis driven, it is worthwhile to look at your data to determine whether there are other interesting findings. Third, if you initially submit your work and it is not particularly well received, do not give up. Remember that the first abstract on the Light criteria was turned down.

WHY THE LIGHT CRITERIA ARE STILL USEFUL

The first reference to use the name the Light criteria that I am aware of was published in 1989.[7] Since the original publication in 1972, there have been many studies comparing other measurements with the Light criteria for the separation of transudates and exudates, but, in general, the Light criteria have been proved to be better than anything else. I am amazed that, after 40 years, the Light criteria are still being used.

Pleural effusions have classically been divided into transudates and exudates. By definition, a transudative pleural effusion develops when the systemic factors influencing the formation or absorption of pleural fluid are altered so that pleural fluid accumulates. The pleural fluid is called a transudate. The permeability of the capillaries to proteins is normal in the area where the fluid is formed. Examples of conditions producing transudative pleural effusions are left ventricular failure producing increased pulmonary interstitial fluid and a resulting pleural effusion, ascites caused by cirrhosis with movement of fluid through the diaphragm, and decreased serum oncotic pressure with hypoproteinemia.[8]

In contrast, an exudative pleural effusion develops when the pleural surfaces or the capillaries in the location where the fluid originates are altered such that fluid accumulates. The most common causes of exudative pleural effusions are pleural malignancy, parapneumonic effusions, and pulmonary embolism.

Why is it important to differentiate transudates from exudates? If a patient has a transudative pleural effusion, then it is only necessary to treat the cause of the effusion, such as heart failure or cirrhosis. However, if it is an exudative effusion, more investigation is indicated to identify the local problem that is causing the pleural effusion.

Why use 2 different measurements to separate transudates from exudates? The pleural fluid/ serum protein ratio is an indication of the permeability of the capillaries in the area where the pleural fluid was formed. In contrast, the pleural fluid LDH level is an indication of the degree of inflammation in the pleural space. Therefore, they measure different things. However, there is no doubt that they are related because inflammation in the pleural space increases the permeability of the capillaries in the pleura.

Why are the Light criteria still useful after 40 years? I think that there are several reasons for its popularity and its usefulness, including (1) it is simple and easy to remember, (2) its measurement is readily available, (3) it is accurate.

Since the Light criteria were first presented, there have been many articles proposing alternatives. One of the measures proposed was the level of cholesterol in the pleural fluid,[9–11] or the ratio of the pleural fluid to the serum cholesterol.[11] The cholesterol measurement is unlikely to be superior to the Light criteria because the pleural fluid cholesterol level can be accurately predicted from the serum cholesterol and the ratio of the pleural fluid to the serum protein level.[12] Cholesterol measurements provide no additional information to the protein ratio. Other proposed measures have included the pleural fluid/serum bilirubin ratio,[13] the pleural fluid viscosity,[14] the level of oxidative stress markers,[15] the level of soluble leukocyte selectin,[16] the level of various cytokines,[17] the level of uric acid,[18] and the pleural fluid/serum cholinesterase ratio.[19] Subsequent articles[20,21] have shown that none of these other measures are superior to the Light criteria in separating transudates from exudates.

When the original article[1] was published, the Light criteria identified all transudates and exudates accurately. However, subsequent studies have shown that the Light criteria classify almost all exudates correctly, but falsely classify about 25% of transudates as exudates. In a study[22] of 249 patients in which there were 185 exudates and 64 transudates, the Light criteria correctly identified 99.5% of exudates but only 75% of transudates. In a recent article,[23] the Light criteria falsely classified 107 of 364 (29%) transudates caused by heart failure and 18 of 102 (18%) transudates caused by hepatic hydrothorax.

Transudates that are falsely classified as exudates usually make exudative criteria by only a slight amount. In an article[23] involving 107 falsely classified transudates, the mean pleural fluid (PF)/ serum protein ratio was 0.51, the mean PF/serum LDH was 0.63, and the mean pleural fluid LDH was 0.34 the upper normal limit for serum for the transudates that were falsely classified. Most transudates are falsely classified by only 1 of the 3 elements of the Light criteria.[23] Most of the patients with transudates who are falsely classified either are receiving diuretics or have a pleural fluid red blood cell (RBC) count greater than $10,000/mm^3$.[24] Romero-Candeira and colleagues[25] performed 3 thoracenteses at 48-hour intervals in 15 patients with pleural effusions caused by heart failure after they were started on diuretics. They reported that the mean pleural fluid protein increased from 2.3 to 3.3 gm/dL and the mean pleural fluid LDH increased from 177 to 288 IU/L. After diuresis, the Light criteria would have classified most of the effusions as exudates.[25]

In the original article,[1] almost all transudates were classified correctly. What is the explanation for the observation that currently about 25% of transudates are falsely classified? I think that there are probably 2 reasons for this discrepancy. First, in the original series, almost all the thoracenteses were done on patients who had just been admitted to the hospital and were not on diuretics. Second, the diuretics are more powerful now than those that were available in 1972, namely hydrochlorothiazide and the mercurial diuretics (ie, mercury chloride; now rarely used).

An alternative approach for the identification of transudates and exudates is to select the cutoff levels that correctly identify the highest percentage of patients. Heffner and colleagues[26] analyzed data from 8 studies with a total of 1448 patients and concluded that the best cutoff levels for the different pleural fluid tests were protein ratio 0.5, LDH ratio 0.45, and LDH 0.45 of the upper limits of normal for serum. The problem with this approach is that some effusions will be misclassified but it is impossible to know whether they are misclassified wrongly as a transudate or an exudate. I still prefer the Light criteria because I want to definitely identify all exudative effusions.

TRANSUDATIVE EFFUSIONS MISCLASSIFIED BY THE LIGHT CRITERIA

When the Light criteria are used, how are those transudative pleural effusions identified that are misclassified? If a patient is clinically suspected of having a transudative effusion but exudative criteria are met by a small margin (protein ratio between 0.5 and 0.65, LDH ratio between 0.6 and 1.0, pleural fluid LDH between two-thirds and the upper normal limit for serum), attempts should be made to determine whether the patient really has a transudative effusion. The 2 main measures that have been proposed to identify these patients are a serum–pleural fluid albumin gradient greater than 1.2 gm/dL or a serum–pleural fluid protein gradient greater than 3.1 gm/dL. Romero-Candeira and colleagues[22] studied 64 patients with transudative pleural effusions and reported that the Light criteria identified 75% correctly, the serum–pleural fluid albumin gradient identified 86% correctly, and the serum–pleural fluid protein gradient identified 91% correctly. In a recent article,[23] 107 of 364 transudates (29%) caused by congestive heart failure (CHF) were misclassified as exudates. In these 107 instances, a serum–pleural fluid protein gradient greater than 3.1 gm/dL identified 55% correctly, whereas a serum–pleural fluid albumin gradient greater than 1.2 gm/dL, which was only performed in 36 patients, identified 83% correctly.[23] In the same report, 18 of 102 transudates (18%) caused by hepatic hydrothorax were misclassified with the Light criteria. The protein gradient and the albumin gradient identified 61% and 62% of these misclassified transudates correctly. An albumin ratio less than 0.6 correctly identified 77% of these transudates caused by hepatic hydrothorax.

My recommendations in view of the 2 studies discussed earlier are as follows. When evaluating a patient who could have a transudative effusion but who meets exudative criteria via the Light criteria by a small margin, I first look at the serum–pleural fluid protein gradient. If this is greater than 3.1 gm/dL, I conclude that the patient has a transudative effusion. I look at the protein gradient first because it is already available from the Light criteria. If this gradient is less than 3.1 gm/dL, I consider measuring the albumin gradient. If the patient may have a hepatic hydrothorax, I measure the albumin ratio. As an alternative, measurement of the serum or pleural fluid N-terminal probrain natriuretic peptide (NT-pro-BNP) can be performed to determine whether the pleural effusion is caused by CHF (discussed than).

Most transudates are caused by CHF. It is preferable to establish the diagnosis of CHF directly. It seems that the diagnosis of CHF as a cause of the pleural effusion can be made with measurement of the NT-pro-BNP in the pleural fluid or the serum. When the ventricles are subjected to increased pressure or volume, NT-pro-BNP and BNP are released into the circulation.[27] The biologically active BNP and the larger NT-pro-BNP are released in equimolar amounts into the circulation.[27]

Porcel and colleagues[28] first showed that the pleural fluid levels of NT-pro-BNP are increased in patients with heart failure. These researchers measured NT-pro-BNP levels in 117 pleural fluid samples with the following diagnosis: CHF, n = 44; malignancy, n = 35; tuberculous pleuritis, n = 20; hepatic hydrothorax, n = 10; and miscellaneous, n = 18. The mean pleural fluid NT-pro-BNP level in the patients with CHF was 6931 pg/mL, which was significantly higher than the 551 pg/mL in patients with hepatic hydrothorax and the 292 pg/mL in patients with exudative pleural effusions.[28] When a cutoff level of 1500 pg/mL was used, the sensitivity was 91% and the specificity was 93% for the diagnosis of CHF.[28] We compared the pleural fluid NT-pro-BNP levels in 10 patients each with effusions caused by CHF, pulmonary embolism, postcoronary artery bypass graft surgery, and malignancy.[29] All the patients with CHF had NT-pro-BNP levels greater than 1500 pg/mL, whereas none of the other patients had NT-pro-BNP levels this high. There have been several subsequent articles evaluating the accuracy of NT-pro-BNP in making the diagnosis of pleural effusion caused by heart failure. In a meta-analysis of 10 studies with a total of 1120 patients, the pooled sensitivity and specificity were 94% and 94% respectively.[30]

There is a close relationship between the levels of NT-pro-BNP in the pleural fluid and serum. Han and colleagues[31] measured the NT-pro-BNP levels in 240 patients and reported that the correlation coefficient between the pleural and serum

NT-pro-BNP was 0.928. In a second study, Kolditz and colleagues[32] measured the serum and pleural fluid NT-pro-BNP levels in 93 patients, including 25 with CHF. They confirmed the results of the study mentioned earlier in that the levels of serum and pleural fluid NT-pro-BNP were closely correlated ($r^2 = 0.90$). In addition, in each of the two studies,[31,32] the values in the pleural fluid and the serum were almost identical. From these latter two studies, it seems that measurement of the pleural fluid NT-pro-BNP levels provides no additional information beyond the serum measurements.

The pleural fluid NT-pro-BNP is also superior to the BNP and the protein gradient in identifying patients with heart failure who meet the Light criteria for exudates.[33] In a study of 20 patients with heart failure who met the Light criteria for exudates, 18 had NT-pro-BNP levels greater than 1300 pg/mL, 16 had NT-pro-BNP levels greater than 1500 pg/mL, but only 10 had a serum–pleural fluid protein gradient greater than 3.1 gm/dL.

The serum or pleural fluid BNP and NT-pro-BNP cannot be used interchangeably in the diagnosis of pleural effusions caused by CHF.[34] The BNP levels are only about 10% of the NT-pro-BNP levels. There is not a close correlation between the BNP levels and the NT-pro-BNP levels ($r = 0.78$).[33,34] Moreover, the diagnostic usefulness of the NT-pro-BNP in making the diagnosis of heart failure is superior to that of the BNP.[33,35]

SUMMARY

The Light criteria serve as a good starting point in the separation of transudates from exudates. The Light criteria misclassify about 25% of transudates as exudates, and most of these patients are on diuretics. If a patient is thought likely to have a disease that produces a transudative pleural effusion but the Light criteria suggest an exudate by only a small margin, the serum–pleural fluid protein gradient should be examined. If this is greater than 3.1 gm/dL, the patient in probably has a transudative effusion. If the gradient is less than 3.1 gm/dL, either the NT-pro-BNP level in the pleural fluid or the serum–pleural fluid albumin gradient can be measured. Either an NT-pro-BNP greater than 1300 pg/mL or an albumin gradient greater than 1.2 gm/dL indicate that the effusion is a transudate.

REFERENCES

1. Light RW, MacGregor MI, Luchsinger PC, et al. Pleural effusions: the diagnostic separation of transudates and exudates. Ann Intern Med 1972;77:507–14.

2. Holten K. Diagnostic value of some biochemical pleural fluid examinations. Scand J Respir Dis Suppl 1968;63:121–5.

3. Wroblewski F, Wroblewski R. The clinical significant of lactic dehydrogenase activity of serous effusions. Ann Intern Med 1958;48:813–22.

4. Light RW, MacGregor MI, Ball WC Jr, et al. Diagnostic significance of pleural fluid pH and PCO_2. Chest 1973;64:591–6.

5. Carr DT, Power MH. Clinical value of measurements of protein in pleural fluid. N Engl J Med 1958;259:926–7.

6. Light RW, MacGregor MI, Ball WC Jr, et al. Pleural fluid lactic acid dehydrogenases and protein content. Ann Intern Med 1972;76:880.

7. Scheurich JW, Keuer SP, Graham DY. Pleural effusion: comparison of clinical judgment and Light's criteria in determining the cause. South Med J 1989;82:1487–91.

8. Light RW. Pleural diseases. 5th edition. Baltimore (MD): Lippincott Williams and Wilkins; 2007.

9. Hamm H, Brohan U, Bohmer R, et al. Cholesterol in pleural effusions: a diagnostic aid. Chest 1987;92:296–302.

10. Valdés L, Pose A, Suarez J, et al. Cholesterol: a useful parameter for distinguishing between pleural exudates and transudates. Chest 1991;99:1097–102.

11. Costa M, Quiroga T, Cruz E. Measurement of pleural fluid cholesterol and lactate dehydrogenase. A simple and accurate set of indicators for separating exudates from transudates. Chest 1995;108:1260–3.

12. Vaz MA, Teixeira LR, Vargas FS, et al. Relationship between pleural fluid and serum cholesterol levels. Chest 2001;119:204–10.

13. Meisel S, Shamiss A, Thaler M, et al. Pleural fluid to serum bilirubin concentration ratio for the separation of transudates from exudates. Chest 1990;98:141–4.

14. Yetkin O, Tek I, Kaya A, et al. A simple laboratory measurement for discrimination of transudative and exudative pleural effusion: pleural viscosity. Respir Med 2006;100:1286–90.

15. Papageorgiou E, Kostikas K, Kiropoulos T, et al. Increased oxidative stress in exudative pleural effusions: a new marker for the differentiation between exudates and transudates? Chest 2005;128:3291–7.

16. Horvath LL, Gallup RA, Worley BD, et al. Soluble leukocyte selectin in the analysis of pleural effusions. Chest 2001;120:362–8.

17. Alexandrakis MG, Kyriakou D, Alexandraki R, et al. Pleural interleukin-1beta in differentiating transudates and exudates: comparative analysis with other biochemical parameters. Respiration 2002;69:201–6.

18. Uzun K, Vural H, Ozer F, et al. Diagnostic value of uric acid to differentiate transudates and exudates. Clin Chem Lab Med 2000;38:661–5.

19. Garcia-Pachon E, Padilla-Navas I, Sanchez JF, et al. Pleural fluid to serum cholinesterase ratio for the separation of transudates and exudates. Chest 1996;110:97–101.
20. Romero S, Candela A, Martin C, et al. Evaluation of different criteria for the separation of pleural transudates from exudates. Chest 1993;104:399–404.
21. Burgess LJ, Maritz FJ, Taljaard JJ. Comparative analysis of the biochemical parameters used to distinguish between pleural transudates and exudates. Chest 1995;107:1604–9.
22. Romero-Candeira S, Hernandez L, Romero-Brufao S, et al. Is it meaningful to use biochemical parameters to discriminate between transudative and exudative pleural effusions? Chest 2002;122:1524–9.
23. Bielsa S, Porcel JM, Castellote J, et al. Solving the Light's criteria misclassification rate of cardiac and hepatic transudates. Respirology 2012;17:721–6.
24. Porcel JM, Esquerda A, Martinez M, et al. Influence of pleural fluid red blood cell count on the misidentification of transudates. Med Clin (Barc) 2008;131:770–2.
25. Romero-Candeira S, Fernandez C, Martin C, et al. Influence of diuretics on the concentration of proteins and other components of pleural transudates in patients with heart failure. Am J Med 2001;110:681–6.
26. Heffner JE, Sahn SA, Brown LK. Multilevel likelihood ratios for identifying exudative pleural effusion. Chest 2002;121:1916–20.
27. Pfister R, Schneider CA. Natriuretic peptides BNP and NT-pro-BNP: established laboratory markers in clinical practice or just perspectives. Clin Chim Acta 2004;349:25–38.
28. Porcel JM, Vives M, Cao G, et al. Measurement of pro-brain natriuretic peptide in pleural fluid for the diagnosis of pleural effusions due to heart failure. Am J Med 2004;116:417–20.
29. Liao H, Na MJ, Dikensoy O, et al. The diagnostic value of pleural fluid NT-proBNP levels in patients with cardiovascular diseases. Respirology 2008;13:53–7.
30. Janda S, Swiston J. Diagnostic accuracy of pleural fluid NT-pro-BNP for pleural effusions of cardiac origin: a systematic review and meta-analysis. BMC Pulm Med 2010;10:58.
31. Han CH, Choi JE, Chung JH. Clinical utility of pleural fluid NT-pro brain natriuretic peptide (NT-proBNP) in patients with pleural effusions. Intern Med 2008;47:1669–74.
32. Kolditz M, Halank M, Schiemanck S, et al. High diagnostic accuracy of NT-proBNP for cardiac origin of pleural effusions. Eur Respir J 2006;28:144–50.
33. Porcel JM, Martínez-Alonso M, Cao G, et al. Biomarkers of heart failure in pleural fluid. Chest 2009;136:671–7.
34. Porcel JM. Utilization of B-type natriuretic peptide and NT-proBNP in the diagnosis of pleural effusions due to heart failure. Curr Opin Pulm Med 2011;17:215–9.
35. Long AC, O'Neal HR Jr, Peng S, et al. Comparison of pleural fluid N-terminal pro-brain natriuretic peptide and brain natriuretic-32 peptide levels. Chest 2010;137:1369–74.

Pleural Fluid Biomarkers
Beyond the Light Criteria

José M. Porcel, MD

KEYWORDS

- Pleural effusion • Biomarkers • Natriuretic peptides • Adenosine deaminase • Tumor markers
- Mesothelin • Fibulin-3 • C-reactive protein

KEY POINTS

- Accurate diagnosis of the cause of a pleural effusion can be challenging.
- Analysis of soluble biomarkers from effusions may be a useful adjunctive.
- Ideal biomarkers should be both sensitive and specific to the disease state being examined and be available at the bedside.
- None of the many reported biomarkers for pleural infection have yet been shown to be more effective than pH in predicting which parapneumonic effusions are complicated.
- The value of pleural fluid tumor markers in diagnosing malignancy remains limited because further pathologic examination is warranted.

The Light criteria have stood the test of time for separating transudates from exudates, a nearly indispensable first step in the evaluation of patients with pleural effusions.[1] The rationale behind this simple initial discrimination is that, if the patient has a transudate, the probable cause is heart failure (HF) or, less commonly, cirrhosis, and the use of diuretics will solve the problem. In contrast, the finding of an exudate widens the differential diagnosis and requires a more precise etiologic search, which may include invasive procedures. Although the Light criteria are extremely sensitive in identifying exudates, they lack specificity in that about 30% and 20% of HF-associated and cirrhosis-associated pleural effusions are misclassified as exudates.[2] Another criticism of the Light criteria is that, other than grouping pleural effusions into transudates and exudates, they do not attach a specific label to a disease. Some experts, including Dr Light, have recommended focusing research on the identification of specific pleural disease markers rather than wasting time and resources in transudate-exudate differentiation.[3]

Hence, moving beyond the Light criteria using effective biomarkers for particular causes may improve clinical management.

A biomarker can be defined as a biological molecule found in blood, other body fluids, or tissues that is a sign of a normal or abnormal process, or of a condition or disease, such as cancer, infection, or HF.[4] Ideal biomarkers are easily measured at a reasonable cost (analytical validity), must provide information that is not already available from a routine clinical assessment (clinical validity), and, eventually, should aid in decision making (clinical usefulness).[4] Although there are many emerging pleural fluid biomarkers under study, few fulfill these 3 criteria well enough to be used clinically. Therefore, this article only discusses those that have consistently shown diagnostic relevance and/or are easily available.

BIOMARKERS OF HF

HF causes more pleural effusions than any other disease. The finding of a transudate by applying

The author has no potential conflicts of interest.
Pleural Diseases Unit, Department of Internal Medicine, Arnau de Vilanova University Hospital, Biomedical Research Institute of Lleida, Avda Alcalde Rovira Roure 80, Lleida 25198, Spain
E-mail address: jporcelp@yahoo.es

Clin Chest Med 34 (2013) 27–37
http://dx.doi.org/10.1016/j.ccm.2012.11.002
0272-5231/13/$ – see front matter © 2013 Elsevier Inc. All rights reserved.

the Light criteria reinforces its diagnosis, because HF accounts for 80% of all transudates. However, HF-related effusions in patients who receive diuretics or have bloody fluids frequently meet the Light exudative criteria by a narrow margin.[5] In addition, differentiating cardiac from noncardiac transudates requires the use of specific disease biomarkers.

Natriuretic Peptides

Natriuretic peptides are neurohormones secreted by the cardiomyocytes in response to stretch and increased pressure in the chambers of the heart.[6] Automated immunometric assays are readily available for brain natriuretic peptide (BNP), the amino-terminal fragment NT-proBNP, and the midregional proatrial natriuretic peptide (MR-proANP). The measurement of BNP or NT-proBNP can be useful in the evaluation of patients presenting in the urgent care setting in whom the clinical diagnosis of HF is uncertain. Patients with a serum BNP level less than 100 pg/mL or NT-proBNP less than 300 pg/mL are unlikely to have HF, whereas those with respective concentrations of more than 500 pg/mL and 450 to 1800 pg/mL (cutoffs depending on and increasing with the patient's age) are likely to have HF.[7] Natriuretic peptides can be detected in pleural fluid using assays originally designed for measuring serum or plasma levels.

Since the first report in 2004,[8] several studies have supported the usefulness of pleural fluid NT-proBNP in determining the cardiac origin of a pleural effusion.[9] In a meta-analysis of 10 publications, totaling 429 cardiac and 691 noncardiac effusions, the test had a pooled sensitivity and specificity of 94%, a likelihood ratio (LR) positive of 15.2, an LR negative of 0.06, a diagnostic odds ratio of 246, and a summary receiver operating characteristic curve of 0.98.[10] In general, LRs of more than 10 or less than 0.1 generate large and usually conclusive shifts from pretest to posttest probability. Therefore, the finding of a pleural fluid NT-proBNP greater than 1500 pg/mL, which is the most commonly reported diagnostic decision threshold,[7] argues convincingly for HF. Moreover, levels less than this cutoff are similarly compelling, decreasing the probability of HF.

Pleural fluid BNP is a less powerful test for decisively determining HF compared with NT-proBNP, as was shown in a head-to-head comparison study (respective areas under the curve [AUC] of 0.90 and 0.96).[11] However, the measurement of pleural fluid MR-proANP has discriminating capacities similar to NT-proBNP.[12] If clinicians choose pleural fluid specimens for natriuretic

peptide testing, the current recommendation is to select NT-proBNP, based on existing evidence and analytical advantages.[7] Several studies have shown a strong correlation between pleural fluid and serum levels of NT-proBNP and comparable operating characteristics at similar or close cutoff values for both.[7,13] As a result, applying the test to serum alone may be sufficient.[14]

In addition, more than 80% of HF-associated effusions that have been misclassified as exudates by the Light criteria exhibit diagnostic levels of NT-proBNP.[5] However, calculating the albumin gradient (serum concentration minus pleural fluid concentration) seems to be equally effective, and simpler, for this purpose.[2] As expected, noncardiac transudates, such as hepatic hydrothoraces, have characteristically low pleural fluid concentrations of natriuretic peptides.[8,11]

BIOMARKERS OF PLEURAL INFECTION

The terms pleural infection and parapneumonic effusions are used interchangeably, although one-fourth of pleural infection cases occur without a concurrent bacterial pneumonia. The typical patient with pleural bacterial infection presents with symptoms of pneumonia (ie, fever, chest pain, dyspnea, cough) along with leukocytosis, raised serum C-reactive protein (CRP) levels, and a chest radiograph showing the effusion and radiological lung infiltrates. However, patients may have a more indolent presentation and several conditions (eg, tuberculosis, connective tissue diseases, pulmonary embolism, pancreatic diseases, or malignancy) can all mimic pleural bacterial infection.

Leukocyte Esterase Reagent Strips

Pleural fluid sampling and analysis are essential to confirm an infection.[15] In a resource-limited health care setting or if biochemistries of the aspirated fluid are not available on an emergency basis, urine reagent strips applied to pleural fluid may expedite diagnostic information. One study tested commercially available reagent strips for leukocyte esterase in the pleural fluid of 42 patients with bacterial infections, 15 with tuberculosis, and 71 with noninfectious causes.[16] A positive test yielded 42% sensitivity, 100% specificity, and an LR positive of 75 for the identification of bacterial infections in the pleural space.

Rapid Pneumococcal Antigen Test

When used in pleural fluid specimens, another quick and simple urinary test, the immunochromatographic detection of the pneumococcal antigen

(Binax NOW *Streptococcus pneumoniae*, Inverness Medical, Scarborough, Maine), allows the etiologic diagnosis of parapneumonic effusions and may help to optimize antimicrobial therapy. One study tested the pneumococcal antigen assay in 140 adult patients with pleural effusions.[17] It was positive in 71% of 34 patients with pneumococcal pneumonia, 7% of 89 nonpneumococcal effusions, and 29% of 17 parapneumonic effusions of unknown microbial cause. Among 28 patients with pneumococcal pneumonia for whom both pleural fluid and urine antigen assays were available, the results were concordant in 18 and discordant in 10 (3 of the 10 had positive tests in pleural fluid and negative in the urine, whereas, in the remaining 7, the opposite occurred).[17] Therefore, ordering a pleural fluid pneumococcal antigen assay is a logical option in patients with parapneumonic effusions and negative urinary tests in which the bacterial cause is being investigated.

CRP

The fluid in parapneumonic effusions is invariably an exudate, with predominantly polymorphonuclear leukocytes in more than 80% of the cases,[15] a feature that is not unique for this condition. Approximately 10%, 20%, and 60% of tuberculous, malignant, and pulmonary emboli–associated pleural fluids, respectively, also reveal neutrophilic predominance.[15] However, if a neutrophilic pleural fluid has CRP concentrations greater than 45 mg/L, it is most likely parapneumonic (LR = 7.7).[18]

More crucial than correctly diagnosing parapneumonic effusions is to identify those of nonpurulent appearance, which require chest drainage (ie, complicated parapneumonic effusions). A delay in implementing the necessary drainage is associated with significant morbidity and mortality. Pleural fluid pH or, alternatively, glucose has a key role in defining complicated parapneumonic effusions.[19] The lower the pH or glucose levels, the more likely the need for pleural drainage. According to existing guidelines, a pH value of less than 7.20 or a glucose less than 60 mg/dL is recommended as an action threshold for chest tube insertion,[20] but decisions should be made on an individual basis. A recent retrospective review that evaluated the capacity of several pleural fluid biochemistries (ie, pH, glucose and CRP) of 340 nonpurulent parapneumonic effusions to discriminate complicated from uncomplicated effusions showed that none could be identified as being superior to the others (all area under the curve ~0.80).[18] Values of pH less than 7.20, glucose <60 mg/dL, and CRP greater than 100 mg/L suggested complicated parapneumonic effusions (positive LRs of 5.5, 5.7, and 5, respectively), but the absence of these findings did not change the probability of complicated effusions sufficiently (all negative LRs ~0.48).[18] As expected, a combination of CRP with either pH or glucose using an Or rule, wherein the pleural space would be drained if any test is positive, increased sensitivity for detecting complicated parapneumonic effusions to about 80%. In contrast, the combination using an And rule, wherein a chest tube would be inserted if both tests were positive, increased the specificity to 97%.[18] Whether pleural fluid CRP may be included among the routine biochemical data used to make decisions on the drainage of nonpurulent infectious collections warrants further study.

Newer Biomarkers of Infection

In addition to the tests described earlier, several promising biomarkers of infection have been used in research, although not in clinical practice.[21] They reflect different stages of the inflammatory cascade triggered by microorganisms and can be measured by commercially available immunoassays. Some reported pleural fluid biomarkers with acceptable performances for discriminating between nonpurulent complicated and uncomplicated parapneumonic effusions are, in decreasing order of positive LRs, tumor necrosis factor α greater than or equal to 80 pg/mL (LR 6.8),[22] myeloperoxidase greater than 3000 μg/L (LR 5.9),[23] matrix metalloproteinase-2 less than or equal to 343 ng/mL (LR 5.5),[24] neutrophil elastase greater than 3500 μg/L (LR 4.6),[25] interleukin-8 greater than or equal to 1000 pg/mL (LR 4.6),[26] lipopolysaccharide-binding protein greater than or equal to 17 μg/mL (LR 4),[27] and soluble triggering receptor expressed on myeloid cell greater than or equal to 180 pg/mL (LR 3.9).[27] Other biomarkers may be clinically meaningful because of their high sensitivity and extremely low LR negative for complicated effusions. Examples are pleural interleukin 1β greater than 3.9 pg/mL (LR negative 0.02),[28] terminal complement complex SC5b-9 greater than 2000 μg/L (LR negative 0.03),[29] and 8-isoprostane greater than 35.1 pg/mL (LR negative 0.04)[30]; values lower than the reported thresholds make a complicated parapneumonic effusion highly unlikely. Procalcitonin, a prohormone used to confirm or exclude the diagnosis of severe bacterial infection, lacks the ability to separate complicated from uncomplicated effusions when evaluated in pleural fluid.[27]

Caveats of Complicated Parapneumonic Marker Studies

Overall, there are several problems when trying to assess the discriminatory properties of biomarker measurements for pleural infection in the published literature.[19,21] First, there is no errorless gold standard for judging whether the physician's decision to insert a chest tube was correct, possibly resulting in a misclassified complicated effusion. Second, an incorporation bias can occur when the clinician makes the diagnosis of a complicated effusion after considering the results of routinely used tests, such as pleural fluid pH (ie, the index test forms part of the reference standard, thereby overestimating its diagnostic accuracy). This bias may partly justify the nonsuperiority of newer laboratory markers compared with traditional ones. In addition, the reported operating characteristics of many investigative biomarkers are based on studies with small sample sizes, which result in wide 95% confidence intervals. Because the new biomarkers provide the same information as the widely established pH and glucose, or the easily performed CRP, it is not anticipated that they will replace or be added to those currently being used for clinical decision making in parapneumonic effusions.

BIOMARKERS OF TUBERCULOSIS

The need for biomarkers in pleural tuberculosis (TB) is justified by the low yield of conventional microbiological studies caused by the paucity of *Mycobacterium tuberculosis* in pleural fluid, and the 6 to 8 weeks required to obtain results. For example, in a retrospective analysis of 214 patients with pleural tuberculosis, solid culture media for mycobacteria were positive in just 28% of sputum and 15% of pleural fluid samples.[31] The respective figures for acid-fast bacilli staining, a more rapid determination technique, were 14% and 3%.[31] Pleural biopsy may show granulomas in approximately 80% of cases, but it is invasive and its yield and complication rate depend on operator skills.[32]

The presence of mycobacterial antigens in the pleural space elicits an intense immune response, initially by neutrophils and subsequently by macrophages and T-lymphocytes, which results in a lymphocyte-predominant exudative effusion. The cell-mediated immune response provokes the release of T-lymphocyte enzymes, such as adenosine deaminase (ADA), and proinflammatory cytokines (eg, γ-interferon [IFN-γ]) into the pleural space. Numerous nonspecific inflammatory and immune response biomarkers have been evaluated diagnostically in tuberculous pleurisy, but none have been found to be superior to pleural fluid ADA or IFN-γ levels.[33]

Adenosine Deaminase

The ADA assay is inexpensive, rapid, simple to perform, and has a pivotal role for the immediate presumptive diagnosis of tuberculous pleuritis. In the largest series from a single center published to date, ADA levels were evaluated in the pleural fluid of 2104 consecutive patients, of whom 221 (10.5%) had tuberculosis.[34] The pleural fluid ADA level exceeded 35 U/L in 93% of pleural tuberculosis. In contrast, only 10% of lymphocytic exudates from patients with other diagnoses had such high levels.[34] These results are similar to those from a meta-analysis of 63 studies that included 2796 patients with tuberculous pleuritis and 5297 with nontuberculous effusions.[35] The reported sensitivity, specificity, positive LR, negative LR, and odds ratio of pleural fluid ADA levels in the diagnosis of pleural tuberculosis were 92%, 90%, 9, 0.10, and 110, respectively.[35] The most widely accepted cutoff value for pleural ADA is 40 U/L. Although one-third of parapneumonic effusions and 70% of empyemas exhibit ADA levels above this threshold, they can be easily distinguished from pleural tuberculosis by the clinical picture, the fluid appearance, and because parapneumonic effusions predominantly have neutrophils in the pleural fluid.[32,34] High pleural fluid ADA levels have also been reported in more than half of lymphomatous effusions.[34] An extremely high ADA activity in pleural fluid (>250 U/L) should raise the suspicion of empyema or lymphoma rather than tuberculosis.[34]

There are 2 different molecular forms of ADA: ADA1 and ADA2. The first is ubiquitous and found in many cells, whereas the second is produced mainly by monocyte/macrophages and is responsible for most of the increase in ADA activity in tuberculous pleural fluids.[32] ADA probably retains its usefulness in patients positive for human immunodeficiency virus with low CD4 cell counts because monocytes are not significantly affected by the retroviral infection.[36] Tuberculous fluids with polymorphonuclear predominance show higher pleural ADA levels, at the expense of both ADA1 and ADA2 isoenzymes, than their lymphocytic counterpart.[31] As a result, the diagnostic performance of ADA is reliable even in the early stage of tuberculous pleuritis.

Pleural fluid ADA is routinely used in the diagnostic work-up in countries where the prevalence of tuberculosis as a cause of exudative effusions is high or moderate. In countries where it is low (eg, 1%), the estimated positive predictive value of the ADA test may be as low as 7%. Even so, the negative predictive value remains high (99.9%).[34] For this reason, ADA can still be used to confidently exclude the disease.

IFN-γ

IFN-γ is a cytokine released by activated CD4+ T lymphocytes and increases the mycobactericidal activity of macrophages. There exist 2 different methods to evaluate it in the pleural fluid. The first is the measurement of unstimulated IFN-γ (most commonly by enzyme-linked immunosorbent assay [ELISA]), and the second consists of the detection of IFN-γ release by pleural fluid mononuclear cells under stimulation with specific antigens of M tuberculosis (IFN-γ–releasing assays [IGRA]). Concerning unstimulated IFN-γ, a meta-analysis of 22 studies that included 782 patients with tuberculous and 1319 with nontuberculous effusions revealed that the mean sensitivity of the test was 89%, the mean specificity was 97%, and maximum joint sensitivity and specificity was 95%.[37] As in the ADA assays, hematologic malignancies and empyemas can cause increased IFN-γ levels in pleural fluid. Studies that have directly compared ADA and IFN-γ in patients with pleural tuberculosis have reported a slightly higher, but nonsignificant, accuracy of the latter.[38] However, because there is little difference in performance between the two and ADA is both cheaper and simpler, ADA is considered to be the preferred test.[32] A major limitation of ADA is that it does not provide culture and drug sensitivity information, which may be vital in countries with a high degree of resistance to antituberculous drugs. A tissue diagnosis with accompanying culture and sensitivity data should be pursued if the patient showing a lymphocytic exudative effusion with a high ADA concentration is from a region with high levels of mycobacterial resistance.

IGRAs were primarily designed to detect latent tuberculosis, but their role in the work-up of suspected tuberculous effusions is now being debated. In a meta-analysis of 7 publications, totaling 213 patients with tuberculous and 153 with nontuberculous effusions, the summary estimates of sensitivity, specificity, positive LR, and negative LR for pleural IGRA assays (T-SPOT-TB and Quanti-FERON-TB) in diagnosing tuberculosis were 75%, 82%, 3.5, and 0.24, respectively.[39] Because IGRAs are technically complex and expensive tests that usually produce an unacceptable number of false-positive and false-negative results, and 15% of cases are limited in their inability to isolate sufficient mononuclear cells to

perform the assay,[40] their regular use cannot be supported.

Nucleic Acid Amplification Tests

Assays for the amplification and detection of M tuberculosis nucleic acids in pleural fluid have high specificity (>95%), but varying and generally disappointingly low sensitivities (~60%) that, in addition to the high cost of the tests, render them inappropriate for ruling the disease in or out in other than investigational settings.[41] In-house nucleic acid amplification tests produce highly inconsistent results compared with those that are commercial and standardized. The low test sensitivity is mainly the result of the technical aspects of nucleic acid extraction, the presence of inhibitors in the pleural fluid, and the paucibacillary nature of the disease.

BIOMARKERS OF MALIGNANCY

The diagnosis of malignant pleural effusions is most easily established by showing malignant cells in the pleural space. However, pleural fluid cytology is positive in only 60% of cases, leading to the need for further diagnostic tests.[15] The cytology is more likely to be positive with adenocarcinoma than squamous cell carcinoma or lymphoma. Moreover, it provides a definitive diagnosis of mesothelioma in only one-third of cases and a suspected diagnosis in a further 20%.[42]

Classic Tumor Markers

Many articles have suggested the possibility of diagnosing pleural malignancy when increased levels of tumor markers in the pleural fluid are found. A myriad of tumor markers have been evaluated. In a systematic review of 45 publications, comprising 2834 patients with malignant and 3251 patients with nonmalignant effusions, the summary estimates of pleural fluid carcinoembryonic antigen (CEA) for identifying the former were sensitivity 54%, specificity 94%, positive LR 9.5, and negative LR 0.49.[43] In an additional meta-analysis by the same investigators, the pooled sensitivity, specificity, positive LR, and negative LR of the following 4 pleural markers for differentiating malignant from benign effusions were cancer antigen (CA) 125, 0.48/0.85/5.9/0.54; CA 15-3, 0.51/0.96/11.7/0.52; CA 19-9, 0.25/0.96/10.4/0.7; and cytokeratin fragment (CYFRA) 21-1 0.55/0.91/6.5/0.43.[44] For tumor markers to be useful diagnostically, selected cutoff points have to be 100% specific. However, the adoption of a cutoff level that is not exceeded by any of the benign effusions generates insensitive tests. For example, one study measured the pleural fluid levels of CEA, CA 15-3, CA 125, and CYFRA 21-1 in 416 patients, including 166 with definitive malignant effusions, 77 with probable malignant effusions, and 173 with benign effusions.[45] When cutoff levels that were 100% specific were selected (ie, CEA>50 ng/mL, CA 15-3 >75 U/mL, CA 125 >2800 U/mL, and CYFRA 21-1 >175 ng/mL), 54% of the malignant effusions were classified as such, and more than one-third of the cytology-negative malignant pleural effusions were identified by at least 1 marker. None of the 22 lymphomas and 7 sarcomas exceeded the cutoff points set by the panel of tumor markers. The same was true for CEA in the 11 mesotheliomas, giving support that high pleural fluid concentrations of CEA are valuable in ruling out this tumor type.[45]

An increased level of some tumor markers in pleural fluid not only suggests malignancy, but is also an independent indicator of life expectancy. In a series of 224 confirmed metastatic pleural malignancies caused by adenocarcinoma or squamous cell carcinoma, those with pleural CA 125 greater than 1000 U/mL and CYFRA 21-1 greater than 100 ng/mL survived 7 months less.[46] The clinical applicability of measuring tumor markers in pleural fluid is limited because, even with high concentrations, further confirmatory cytohistologic diagnosis is necessary.

Mesothelin

Mesothelioma can be difficult to diagnose. Cytologic examination of the pleural fluid often shows equivocal results, and international guidelines do not recommend it as the sole pathologic method.[47] Thoracoscopic biopsy provides the most accurate definitive diagnosis. The search for a single diagnostic marker of mesothelioma has so far been evasive. Mesothelin, a 40 kDa membrane-bound protein attached to the mesothelial cell surface by phosphatidylinositol, has been the most extensively investigated.[48] It can be measured by ELISA in either serum or pleural fluid.

An individual patient data meta-analysis of 4491 patients, among whom there were 1026 with malignant mesothelioma (MM), examined the accuracy of serum mesothelin in the diagnosis of mesothelioma.[49] When applying a common threshold of 2 nmol/L, the summary estimate sensitivity was 47% and specificity was 96%. The use of mesothelin in early diagnosis was evaluated for differentiating 217 patients with stage I or II epithelioid and biphasic mesothelioma from 1612 symptomatic or high-risk controls.[49] At

a specificity of 95%, approximately 70% of patients with early mesothelioma would have remained undetected. This unacceptably low sensitivity limits the use of mesothelin in early diagnosis. Serum mesothelin has also been suggested as a complementary tool for detecting tumor progression and evaluating response to treatment,[50–52] although it has not yet been implemented in routine clinical practice for this purpose.

Similar to serum mesothelin, pleural fluid mesothelin levels are increased in patients with mesothelioma relative to levels in effusions from other causes. In several studies, pleural mesothelin has yielded approximately 65% sensitivity, 90% specificity, positive LR of 7, and AUC greater than 0.80 for discriminating between mesothelioma and other malignancies or nonmalignant diseases.[53–57] Different accuracies in various reports may have been influenced by the proportion of sarcomatoid mesotheliomas (which do not express mesothelin), or the type of effusions in the nonmesothelioma groups (eg, mesothelin is increased in ovarian and pancreatic cancer). In general, pleural mesothelin levels greater than 20 nM strongly suggest mesothelioma. In one study of 105 cytology-negative effusions, 9 (60%) of 15 mesotheliomas had pleural fluid mesothelin concentrations above this threshold, in contrast with only 3 (3%) of 90 nonmesothelioma effusions.[56] Although the use of pleural mesothelin as a biomarker may reinforce the suspicion of mesothelioma, histopathologic diagnosis remains the gold standard.

Fibulin-3

Fibulin-3 is an extracellular glycoprotein that mediates cell-to-cell interactions and has variable angiogenic effects. In a unique prospective study that included a subsequent blinded validation cohort, pleural fluid fibulin-3 levels were measured by using a commercially available ELISA in 74 patients with mesothelioma, 39 with benign effusions, and 54 with nonmesothelioma malignant effusions.[58] At the best cutoff value of greater than 346 ng/mL, fibulin-3 discriminated mesothelioma effusions from those with other causes with 84% sensitivity, 92% specificity, LR positive of 11, LR negative of 0.17, and AUC of 0.93. If confirmed in future studies, this biomarker will become a useful addition to the mesothelioma diagnostic process.

Immunocytochemical Markers

In the examination of pleural fluid, a cytomorphologic distinction between reactive mesothelial cells, MM, and metastatic adenocarcinoma can often be difficult because of significant overlapping cytologic features. Immunocytochemical staining on cell block preparations assists in establishing such discriminations through the application of panels consisting of a variety of antibodies (**Table 1**).[59] However, there is no agreement on the ideal antibody combination, but a sensitivity of about 80% is desirable for inclusion in the panel.[60]

To confidently validate the diagnosis of epithelioid mesothelioma as opposed to adenocarcinoma, 2 positive mesothelioma markers along with 2 negative adenocarcinoma markers are required (**Table 1**).[47] The panel can be expanded if the results are inconclusive. This author's recommendation is to initially use small panels, which include epithelial membrane antigen (EMA), calretinin, CEA, and thyroid transcription factor-1 (TTF-1).[61–63]

Another indication for effusion immunocytochemistry is to establish the primary site of a malignant effusion in patients with an occult primary or multiple primaries. For example, determination of the primary origin of adenocarcinomas, the most commonly found malignancy in effusion samples, may necessitate the use of the following immunocytochemical markers: TTF-1 (lung cancer), cytokeratin 7 (upper gastrointestinal and pancreatobiliary tract), cytokeratin 20 (colorectal) and, in female patients, estrogen receptors (breast, female genital tract), mammaglobin (breast), and Wilms tumor gene 1 (WT-1; female genital tract).[59]

Different molecular tests, such as fluorescent in situ hybridization and gene expression, may complement cytology in diagnosing malignant effusions, but require specialized equipment and personnel, which limits their introduction into routine clinical practice.[64]

Table 1
Immunocytochemical profile for differentiating between benign and malignant effusions[a]

Marker	Reactive Mesothelial Cells	Mesothelioma	Adenocarcinoma
Markers of Malignancy			
EMA (clone E29)	Negative	Positive	Positive
GLUT-1	Negative	Positive	Positive
Mesothelial Markers			
Desmin	Positive	Negative	Negative
Calretinin	Positive	Positive	Negative
CK 5/6	Positive	Positive	Negative
WT-1	Positive	Positive	Negative[b]
Mesothelin	Positive	Positive	Negative
HBME-1	Positive	Positive	Negative
Podoplanin	Positive	Positive	Negative
D2-40	Positive	Positive	Negative
Carcinoma Markers			
CEA	Negative	Negative	Positive
MOC-31	Negative	Negative	Positive
Ber-EP4	Negative	Negative	Positive
Leu-M1 (CD15)	Negative	Negative	Positive
B72.3	Negative	Negative	Positive
BG8 (Lewis)	Negative	Negative	Positive
TTF-1	Negative	Negative	Positive[c]
Napsin A	Negative	Negative	Positive[d]
Estrogen receptor (ER-1D5)	Negative	Negative	Positive[e]

[a] These are the expected results, but there may be deviations between cases.
[b] Except in ovarian cancer.
[c] Only in non–squamous cell lung and thyroid cancers.
[d] In lung adenocarcinomas and renal cell carcinomas.
[e] Only in breast and female genital tract carcinomas.

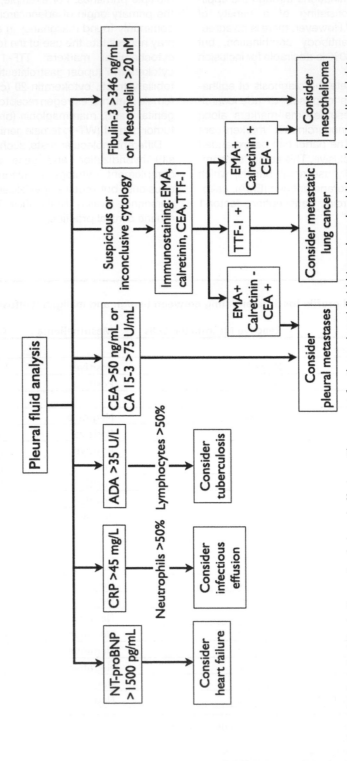

Fig. 1. Biomarker-based etiologic diagnosis of pleural effusions. The request for these pleural fluid biomarkers should be guided by clinical data.

SUMMARY

Accurate diagnosis of the cause of a pleural effusion can be challenging. Analysis of soluble biomarkers from effusions may be a useful adjunctive.[47] Ideal biomarkers should be sensitive and specific to the disease state being examined, and available at the bedside. These characteristics are met by the natriuretic peptide NT-proBNP and the enzyme ADA. Pleural fluid NT-proBNP levels more than 1500 pg/mL are practically diagnostic of HF, whereas an ADA activity greater than 35 to 40 U/L in the pleural fluid provides strong evidence for tuberculosis. None of the many reported biomarkers for pleural infection have yet been shown to be more effective than pH in predicting which parapneumonic effusions are complicated. The value of pleural fluid tumor markers in diagnosing malignancy remains limited because further pathologic examination is warranted. In patients with effusions of undetermined cause and negative cytology, an increased pleural fluid mesothelin or fibulin-3 level strongly favors, although it is not definitive of, mesothelioma. Immunocytochemistry is essential for the diagnosis of mesothelioma and should be applied as a panel of antibodies on cell block sections, including at least 2 mesothelial cell markers and 2 other appropriate antibodies for the alternative pathology being considered, either reactive mesothelial cells or metastatic adenocarcinoma. A suggested algorithm for the investigation of pleural effusions, based on the inclusion of widely available and evidence-supported biomarkers, is shown in **Fig. 1**.

REFERENCES

1. Porcel JM, Light RW. Diagnostic approach to pleural effusion in adults. Am Fam Physician 2006;73:1211–20.
2. Bielsa S, Porcel JM, Castellote J, et al. Solving the Light's criteria misclassification rate of cardiac and hepatic transudates. Respirology 2012;17:721–6.
3. Gary Lee YC, Davies RJ, Light RW. Diagnosing pleural effusion: moving beyond transudate-exudate separation. Chest 2007;131:942–3.
4. Henry NL, Hayes DF. Cancer biomarkers. Mol Oncol 2012;6:140–6.
5. Porcel JM. Pleural effusions from congestive heart failure. Semin Respir Crit Care Med 2010;31:689–97.
6. Porcel JM. The use of probrain natriuretic peptide in pleural fluid for the diagnosis of pleural effusions resulting from heart failure. Curr Opin Pulm Med 2005;11:329–33.
7. Porcel JM. Utilization of BNP and NT-proBNP in the diagnosis of pleural effusions due to heart failure. Curr Opin Pulm Med 2011;17:215–9.
8. Porcel JM, Vives M, Cao G, et al. Measurement of pro-brain natriuretic peptide in pleural fluid for the diagnosis of pleural effusions due to heart failure. Am J Med 2004;116:417–20.
9. Zhou Q, Ye ZJ, Su Y, et al. Diagnostic value of N-terminal pro-brain natriuretic peptide for pleural effusion due to heart failure: a meta-analysis. Heart 2010;96:1207–11.
10. Janda S, Swiston J. Diagnostic accuracy of pleural fluid NT-pro-BNP for pleural effusions of cardiac origin: a systematic review and meta-analysis. BMC Pulm Med 2010;10:58.
11. Porcel JM, Martínez-Alonso M, Cao G, et al. Biomarkers of heart failure in pleural fluid. Chest 2009;136:671–7.
12. Porcel JM, Bielsa S, Morales JL, et al. Comparison of pleural fluid NT-proBNP, MR-proANP and MR-proADM for the diagnosis of cardiac effusions. Respirology, in press.
13. Porcel JM, Chorda J, Cao G, et al. Comparing serum and pleural fluid pro-brain natriuretic peptide (NT-proBNP) levels with pleural-to-serum albumin gradient for the identification of cardiac effusions misclassified by Light's criteria. Respirology 2007;12:654–9.
14. Hooper C, Lee YC, Maskell N. BTS Pleural Guideline Group. Investigation of a unilateral pleural effusion in adults: British Thoracic Society pleural disease guideline 2010. Thorax 2010;65(Suppl 2):ii4–17.
15. Porcel JM. Pearls and myths in pleural fluid analysis. Respirology 2011;16:44–52.
16. Porcel JM, Esquerda A, Bielsa S. A specific point of care screen for infectious effusions using reagent strips. Eur Respir J 2011;37:1528–30.
17. Porcel JM, Ruiz-González A, Falguera M, et al. Contribution of a pleural antigen assay (Binax NOW) to the diagnosis of pneumococcal pneumonia. Chest 2007;131:1442–7.
18. Porcel JM, Bielsa S, Esquerda A, et al. Pleural fluid C-reactive protein contributes to the diagnosis and assessment of severity of parapneumonic effusions. Eur J Intern Med 2012;23:447–50.
19. Tobin CL, Porcel JM, Wrightson JM, et al. Diagnosis of pleural infection: state of the art. Curr Respir Care Rep 2012;1:101–10.
20. Davies HE, Davies RJO, Davies CWH. Management of pleural infection in adults: British Thoracic Society pleural disease guideline 2010. Thorax 2010;65(Suppl 2):ii41–53.
21. Porcel JM. Pleural fluid tests to identify complicated parapneumonic effusions. Curr Opin Pulm Med 2010;16:357–61.
22. Porcel JM, Vives M, Esquerda A. Tumour necrosis factor-α in pleural fluid: a marker of complicated parapneumonic effusions. Chest 2004;125:160–4.
23. Alegre J, Jufresa J, Segura R, et al. Pleural-fluid myeloperoxidase in complicated and noncomplicated parapneumonic effusions. Eur Respir J 2002;19:320–5.

24. Oikonomidi S, Kostikas K, Kalomenidis I, et al. Matrix metalloproteinase levels in the differentiation of parapneumonic pleural effusions. Respiration 2010;80: 285–91.

25. Alemán C, Alegre J, Segura RM, et al. Polymorphonuclear elastase in the early diagnosis of complicated pyogenic pleural effusions. Respiration 2003;70:462–7.

26. Porcel JM, Galindo C, Esquerda A, et al. Pleural fluid interleukin-8 and C-reactive protein for discriminating complicated non-purulent from uncomplicated parapneumonic effusions. Respirology 2008; 13:58–62.

27. Porcel JM, Vives M, Cao G, et al. Biomarkers of infection in pleural fluid for the differential diagnosis of pleural effusions. Eur Respir J 2009;34:1383–9.

28. Marchi E, Vargas FS, Acencio MM, et al. Pro- and anti-inflammatory cytokines levels in complicated and non-complicated parapneumonic effusions. Chest 2012;141:183–9.

29. Vives M, Porcel JM, Gázquez I, et al. Pleural SC5b-9: a test for identifying complicated parapneumonic effusions. Respiration 2000;67:433–8.

30. Tsilioni I, Kostikas K, Kalomenidis I, et al. Diagnostic accuracy of biomarkers of oxidative stress in parapneumonic pleural effusions. Eur J Clin Invest 2011;41:349–56.

31. Bielsa S, Palma S, Pardina M, et al. Comparison of polymorphonuclear- and lymphocytic-rich tuberculous pleural effusions. Int J Tuberc Lung Dis 2013; 17:85–9.

32. Porcel JM. Tuberculous pleural effusion. Lung 2009; 187:263–70.

33. Trajman A, Pai M, Dheda K, et al. Novel tests for diagnosing tuberculous pleural effusion: what works and what does not? Eur Respir J 2008;31:1098–106.

34. Porcel JM, Esquerda A, Bielsa S. Diagnostic performance of adenosine deaminase activity in pleural fluid: a single-center experience with over 2100 consecutive patients. Eur J Intern Med 2010;21: 419–23.

35. Liang QL, Shi HZ, Wang K, et al. Diagnostic accuracy of adenosine deaminase in tuberculous pleurisy: a meta-analysis. Respir Med 2008;102: 744–54.

36. Baba K, Hoosen AA, Langeland N, et al. Adenosine deaminase activity is a sensitive marker for the diagnosis of tuberculous pleuritis in patients with very low CD4 counts. PLoS One 2008;3:e2788.

37. Jiang J, Shi HZ, Liang QL, et al. Diagnostic value of interferon-gamma in tuberculous pleurisy: a meta-analysis. Chest 2007;131:1133–41.

38. Kalantri Y, Hemvani N, Chitnis DS. Evaluation of real-time polymerase chain reaction, interferon-gamma, adenosine deaminase, and immunoglobulin A for the efficient diagnosis of pleural tuberculosis. Int J Infect Dis 2011;15:e226–31.

39. Zhou Q, Chen YQ, Qin SM, et al. Diagnostic accuracy of T-cell interferon-γ release assays in tuberculous pleurisy: a meta-analysis. Respirology 2011;16: 473–80.

40. Dheda K, van Zyl-Smit RN, Sechi LA, et al. Utility of quantitative T-cell responses versus unstimulated interferon-γ for the diagnosis of pleural tuberculosis. Eur Respir J 2009;34:1118–26.

41. Pai M, Flores LL, Hubbard A, et al. Nucleic acid amplification tests in the diagnosis of tuberculous pleuritis: a systematic review and meta-analysis. BMC Infect Dis 2004;4:6.

42. Rakha EA, Patil S, Abdulla K, et al. The sensitivity of cytologic evaluation of pleural fluid in the diagnosis of malignant mesothelioma. Diagn Cytopathol 2010;38:874–9.

43. Hsi HZ, Liang QL, Jiang J, et al. Diagnostic value of carcinoembryonic antigen in malignant pleural effusion: a meta-analysis. Respirology 2008;13:518–27.

44. Liang QL, His HZ, Qin XJ, et al. Diagnostic accuracy of tumour markers for malignant pleural effusion: a meta-analysis. Thorax 2008;63:35–41.

45. Porcel JM, Vives M, Esquerda A, et al. Use of a panel of tumor markers (carcinoembryonic antigen, cancer antigen 125, carbohydrate antigen 15-3, and cytokeratin 19 fragments) in pleural fluid for the differential diagnosis of benign and malignant effusions. Chest 2004;126:1757–63.

46. Bielsa S, Esquerda A, Salud A, et al. High levels of tumor markers in pleural fluid correlate with poor survival in patients with adenocarcinomatous or squamous malignant effusions. Eur J Intern Med 2009;20:383–6.

47. Scherpereel A, Astoul P, Baas P, et al. Guidelines of the European Respiratory Society and the European Society of Thoracic Surgeons for the management of malignant pleural mesothelioma. Eur Respir J 2010; 35:479–95.

48. Tung A, Bilaceroglu S, Porcel JM, et al. Biomarkers in pleural diseases. US Respir Dis 2011;7:26–31.

49. Hollevoet K, Reitsma JB, Creaney J, et al. Serum mesothelin for diagnosing malignant pleural mesothelioma: an individual patient data meta-analysis. J Clin Oncol 2012;30:1541–9.

50. Creaney J, Francis RJ, Dick IM, et al. Serum soluble mesothelin concentrations in malignant pleural mesothelioma: relationship to tumor volume, clinical stage and changes in tumor burden. Clin Cancer Res 2011;17:1181–9.

51. Hollevoet K, Nackaerts K, Gosselin R, et al. Soluble mesothelin, megakaryocyte potentiating factor, and osteopontin as markers of patient response and outcome in mesothelioma. J Thorac Oncol 2011;6: 1930–7.

52. Franko A, Dolzan V, Kovac V, et al. Soluble mesothelin-related peptide levels in patients with malignant mesothelioma. Dis Markers 2012;32:123–31.

53. Scherpereel A, Grigoriu B, Conti M, et al. Soluble mesothelin-related peptides in the diagnosis of malignant pleural mesothelioma. Am J Respir Crit Care Med 2006;173:1155–60.

54. Creaney J, Yeoman D, Naumoff LK, et al. Soluble mesothelin in effusions: a useful tool for the diagnosis of malignant mesothelioma. Thorax 2007;62:569–76.

55. Alemán C, Porcel JM, Segura RM, et al. Pleural fluid mesothelin for the differential diagnosis of exudative pleural effusions. Med Clin (Barc) 2009;133:449–53.

56. Davies HE, Sadler RS, Bielsa S, et al. Clinical impact and reliability of pleural fluid mesothelin in undiagnosed pleural effusions. Am J Respir Crit Care Med 2009;180:437–44.

57. Fujimoto N, Gemba K, Asano M, et al. Soluble mesothelin-related protein in pleural effusion from patients with malignant pleural mesothelioma. Exp Ther Med 2010;1:313–7.

58. Pass HI, Levin SM, Harbut MR, et al. Fibulin-3 as a blood and effusion biomarker for pleural mesothelioma. N Engl J Med 2012;367:1417–27.

59. Ganjei-Azar P, Jordà M, Krishan A. Effusion cytology. A practical guide to cancer diagnosis. New York: Demos Medical; 2011.

60. Zeren EH, Demirag F. Benign and malignant mesothelial proliferation. Surg Pathol 2010;3: 83–107.

61. van der Bij S, Schaake E, Koffijberg H, et al. Markers for the non-invasive diagnosis of mesothelioma: a systematic review. Br J Cancer 2011;104: 1325–33.

62. Betta PG, Magnani C, Bensi T, et al. Immunohistochemistry and molecular diagnostics of pleural malignant mesothelioma. Arch Pathol Lab Med 2012;136:253–61.

63. Porcel JM. Immunocytochemical markers for metastatic lung adenocarcinoma. Int Pleural Newsl 2012;10:8–9. Available at: http://www.musc.edu/pleuralnews/IPN/.

64. Sriram KB, Relan V, Clarke BE, et al. Diagnostic molecular biomarkers for malignant pleural effusions. Future Oncol 2011;7:737–52.

Defying Gravity
Subdiaphragmatic Causes of Pleural Effusions

Kyle Bramley, MD[a], Jonathan T. Puchalski, MD, MEd[b],*

KEYWORDS

- Pleural effusions • Peritoneal flow • Lymphatic drainage • Pancreaticopleural fistula
- Yellow nail syndrome

KEY POINTS

- Intra-abdominal fluid may migrate readily into the pleural space through naturally occurring holes in the diaphragm or intradiaphragmatic lymphatics.
- Although any type of fluid in the abdomen may migrate, additional pathologic mechanisms are involved in the development of chylous ascites/chylothorax, yellow nail syndrome, urinothorax, pancreaticopleural fistulas, or other connections.
- In the differential diagnosis of the large list of potential pleural fluid causes, intra-abdominal sources should be entertained by the practicing physician in the right clinical context.

Pleural effusions affect 1.5 million people per year in the United States.[1] The most common cause of transudates is congestive heart failure, whereas the most common causes of exudates include infections and malignancy. Pleural effusions may arise from subdiaphragmatic processes because of the presence of peritoneopleural connections. In pathologic states, increased intra-abdominal fluid promotes additional unidirectional flow of fluid from the abdomen into the thorax and, on occasion, new fistulae may form. In this section, the authors hope to highlight the pathologic subdiaphragmatic processes that cause pleural effusions and explain the basis behind the formation of this type of pleural disease.

NORMAL PERITONEAL FLUID FLOW AND LYMPHATIC DRAINAGE

Fluid, cells, or both can pass from the peritoneal cavity into the pleural space by 2 routes: inherent diaphragmatic holes (either microscopic or macroscopic) or transdiaphragmatic lymphatic vessels. Autopsy examinations have demonstrated that fluid may pass from the peritoneum into the pleura through blebs, representing stretched pleura and herniated peritoneum, at the site of the diaphragmatic defects. Flow is exclusively unidirectional, which is likely because of the normal pressure gradient.[2] Furthermore, the diaphragm, via its lymphatic channels, serves as the main drainage system for the absorption of fluid from the peritoneal cavity into the systemic circulation. Only a small amount of peritoneal fluid actually diffuses into peritoneal blood vessels. Fluid enters subperitoneal lymphatic lacunae through stomata located between mesothelial cells of the peritoneum. The fluid then traverses the diaphragm via its intrinsic lymphatics to reach a series of collecting lymphatics on the diaphragmatic pleura. Although there are 4 pathways for lymphatic drainage from the diaphragm, most goes cranially via retrosternal

The authors declare no conflicts of interest.

[a] Division of Pulmonary, Critical Care and Sleep Medicine, Department of Internal Medicine, Yale University School of Medicine, 15 York Street, LCI 105, New Haven, CT 06510, USA; [b] Division of Pulmonary, Critical Care and Sleep Medicine, Department of Internal Medicine, Yale University School of Medicine, 15 York Street, LCI 100, New Haven, CT 06510, USA

* Corresponding author.

E-mail address: Jonathan.puchalski@yale.edu

Clin Chest Med 34 (2013) 39–46
http://dx.doi.org/10.1016/j.ccm.2012.12.004
0272-5231/13/$ – see front matter © 2013 Elsevier Inc. All rights reserved.

trunks and gets filtered through the parathymic lymph nodes. The drainage then enters the upper terminal thoracic duct or right lymphatic duct. As such, most fluid from the peritoneal space is not transported in the thoracic duct itself.[3]

In contrast to these lymphatic channels for peritoneal fluid, lymph from much of the subdiaphragmatic intravascular structures enters the thoracic duct. The cisterna chyli is an abdominal confluence of lymphatic trunks that receives lymph from the lower extremities, intra-abdominal organs, kidneys, and abdominal wall. This group of channels is generally found at the level of the second lumbar vertebrae (L2) and to the right of the aorta. The thoracic duct starts at the superior pole of the cisterna chyli, traverses the aortic hiatus of the diaphragm, and ascends along the posterior mediastinum. It is right of the midline and lies posterior to the esophagus, between the azygous vein and aorta. It ultimately crosses left of the midline at approximately the level of the fifth thoracic vertebrae where it traverses superiorly behind the aorta and left carotid to enter the neck (**Fig. 1**). The lymph in the thoracic duct enters the blood stream at the junction of the left subclavian and internal jugular veins.[4] Because of the thoracic pressures and the presence of unidirectional flow, the flow through the thoracic duct is unidirectional.

ABNORMAL PERITONEAL FLUID FLOW AND LYMPHATIC DISRUPTION

Various intra-abdominal inflammatory and noninflammatory processes produce fluid on both sides

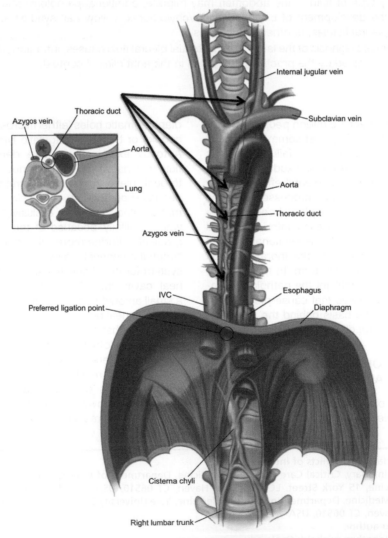

Fig. 1. The normal course of the thoracic duct is highlighted by arrows. IVC, inferior vena cava. (*From* Hematti H, Mehran RJ. Anatomy of the thoracic duct. Thorac Surg Clin 2011;21(2):229–38, ix; with permission.)

of the diaphragm. When excess fluid exists in the peritoneum and normal absorptive routes are overwhelmed, fluid may enter the pleural space via the direct peritoneopleural connections described earlier. This fluid may contain simple ascites arising from portal hypertension, malignant cells (malignant ascites), blood (hemoperitoneum), pus, or other types of fluid. Any intra-abdominal organ may be implicated in causing associated effusions. Tense ascites may cause the diaphragm to stretch and enlarge the preexisting defects, creating a route for conditions, such as hepatic hydrothorax and peritoneal dialysis–associated pleural effusions.

A pleural effusion that develops in patients with cirrhosis, in the absence of cardiopulmonary disease but the presence of portal hypertension, is termed a hepatic hydrothorax. Hepatic hydrothorax develops in 6% of patients with cirrhosis or may occur in patients solely with portal hypertension. With increased abdominal pressure caused by ascites, the normal diaphragmatic gaps may herniate into the pleural cavity, producing pleuroperitoneal blebs. Although typically less than 1 cm in size, they may rupture and provide a free communication between the abdomen and pleural space. They occur more on the right than the left because the left diaphragm seems to be more muscular. A transjugular intrahepatic shunt (TIPS) is the procedure of choice for patients that are not transplant candidates. Thoracentesis may provide symptomatic relief. Pleurodesis may work, although less often than in malignant disease. Thoracoscopic repair of diaphragmatic defects may be considered.[5]

Massive hydrothorax complicating peritoneal dialysis occurs in approximately 3% to 6% of patients. It has been demonstrated by peritoneopleural scintigraphy with a technetium-labeled sulfur colloid (Tc 99m SC) injected into the peritoneal space and followed by serial imaging. Like other peritoneal fluid, it has been reported to be unidirectional. Treatment typically involves the cessation of peritoneal dialysis, although the diaphragmatic defects may also be surgically closed (**Fig. 2**).[6]

Other intra-abdominal pathologic processes may cause excess peritoneal fluid and the resultant pleural disease. For example, an abscess associated with the liver, spleen, gallbladder, appendix, or other intra-abdominal organs may have associated pleural effusions that look like an empyema. The genitourinary system may be associated with pleural effusions, including the kidney, uterus, and ovary. Urinothorax (kidney) is described later. Catamenial hemothorax or pneumothorax likely results from transdiaphragmatic migration of cells that typically line the uterus; bleeding or pneumothorax occur because of hormonal flux at menses. Several conditions associated with the ovary may cause ascites and, hence, pleural disease. These conditions include ovarian cancer (up to 70% may have cytologic ascites), abdominopelvic primary tuberculosis, ovarian hyperstimulation syndrome from assisted reproductive techniques, Meig (benign ovarian tumors) or Pseudo-Meigs syndrome (benign tumors of other organs, including uterus or fallopian tubes), and endometriosis.[7] Of course, any intra-abdominal malignant process may potentially metastasize to the pleural space.

The rest of this review describes subdiaphragmatic processes that have unique anatomic abnormalities that cause pleural disease, including chylothorax, urinothorax, and pancreaticopleural fistulae.

Chylothorax

Although most effusions are yellow, serosanguinous, bloody, or cloudy, other pleural fluid colors and consistency may be found. After excluding pus (empyema) in milky- or white-appearing effusions, chylous or pseudochylous effusions should be considered.

Chyle is formed after digesting food via cells of the small intestine. These enterocytes create

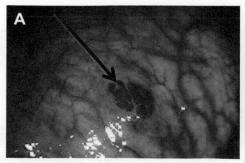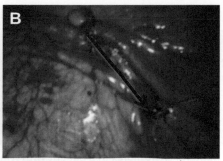

Fig. 2. (*A*) A diaphragmatic defect (*arrow*) seen in the case of peritoneal dialysis-associated hydrothorax. (*B*) This defect was surgically repaired and the diaphragmatic sutures are shown (*arrow*).

chylomicrons that contain triglycerides, phospholipids, cholesterol, and proteins. From the intestinal cells, the molecules move into the abdominal lymphatic system and then into the thoracic duct, as described earlier. When the abdominal lymphatics, cistern chyli, or thoracic duct are disrupted, chylous ascites or chylothorax may result.

Chylous ascites results from anything that obstructs the lymphatic channels in the abdomen, including malignancy (lymphoma, metastatic malignancies, Wilm's tumor), abdominal surgeries (aortic repair, nephrectomy, others), infections in the abdomen (tuberculosis), or forms of cardiac disease (constrictive pericarditis with elevated venous pressure and lymphatic stasis).[4] Because of the aforementioned diaphragmatic holes, chylous ascites may secondarily cause the accumulation of chyle in the thorax (chylothorax).

In addition to upward migration of ascites, various causes are responsible for the formation of a chylothorax. Anatomic variants of the thoracic duct can be present; depending on the level of injury or obstruction, a chylothorax may develop on the right or left side. Chylous effusions are usually the result of trauma (thoracic damage or accidental surgical ligation of the thoracic duct from procedures, such as esophagectomy, coronary artery bypass grafting, lobectomy, neck dissection, and others) or tumor, although miscellaneous or unknown causes occur.[8] Non-Hodgkin lymphoma is the most common malignant cause of chylous effusions. Approximately 38% are related to surgery; 32% to malignancy; 10% are idiopathic; and the remaining 20% are from miscellaneous causes, including granulomatous diseases, radiation, trauma, and lymphatic abnormalities. The thoracic duct may also be dilated by right heart failure and by cirrhosis with portal hypertension. In either condition, chylothorax or chylous ascites may form.

As noted earlier, chylous effusions are often milky, although this gross appearance may also be seen in empyema, cholesterol effusions, or extravascular migration of central venous catheters with lipid infusions. **Fig. 3** demonstrates the varied appearance of chylothorax and chylous ascites.

Less than half of chylous effusions are milky, and most effusions are serous or serosanguinous. Chylothoraces are usually protein-discordant, lymphocyte-predominant exudates (high protein and low lactate dehydrogenase [LDH]). The diagnosis of chylothorax is made by identifying triglycerides in the pleural fluid, with a level of 110 mg/dL or more ($\geq$1.24 mmol/L) considered diagnostic. It is virtually excluded with a level of less than 50 mg/dL (<0.56 mmol/L). Levels between 50 and 100 mg/dL are seen in up to 30% of chylothoraces.[8] The diagnosis can be confirmed by the presence of chylomicrons in the pleural fluid, as demonstrated by electrophoresis.

As described earlier, various conditions can cause chylothorax. The location of leakage from the thoracic duct may be ascertained by lymphoscintigraphy with radiolabeled albumin, dextran, or Tc 99m SC. These labeled colloids generate morphologic and functional imaging data about the lymphatic system. Alternatively, a more invasive lymphangiogram may be performed. It requires cannulation of the lymphatic system and may cause fat embolism to the lungs, hypersensitivity pneumonitis, local tissue necrosis, or worsening lymphedema caused by the contrast. Because these often do not change management and because they are not often available in many medical centers, most patients do not undergo imaging for precise localization of the leak.[9]

Treatment includes pleural drainage, correction of the underlying problem, or reduction in chyle production. Chyle production can be reduced by a low-fat diet rich in medium chain fatty acids. Alternatively, total parenteral nutrition (TPN) can optimize nutrition while bypassing the stomach and intestine. There are also several case reports and case series suggesting a possible role of somatostatin or its synthetic analogue, octreotide, to decrease chyle flow and absorption of lipids.[10]

In some patients, conservative therapy alone may not be sufficient and more invasive management

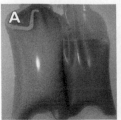 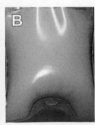 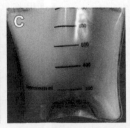 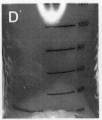 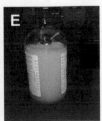

Fig. 3. (A) Bilateral chylothorax in a patient with lymphoma. (B–D) The varying gross appearance of some chylothoraces, in part dependent on the amount of chyle in the fluid. (E) The gross appearance of a patient with chylous ascites.

is necessary. Thoracentesis, chest tubes, tunneled catheters, and pleurodesis are discussed elsewhere in this issue by Sachdeva and colleagues; Mahmood and Wahidi; Myers and Michaud; Lee and Colt. Case series have suggested that thoracoscopy with talc pleurodesis can be a successful minimally invasive approach in nonsurgical patients who are refractory to treatment of the underlying cause.[11] In one retrospective series, medical management and pleurodesis were successful in managing approximately two-thirds of patients, although approximately half of the patients who had postoperative chylothoraces required surgical intervention. In this series, high output (greater than 1 L/d) was the best predictor of the need for surgical intervention.[12] Surgical therapy generally consists of either video-assisted thoracoscopic surgery or thoracotomy with ligation of the thoracic duct.

Care should be taken to distinguish chylous effusions from pseudochylous effusions, otherwise known as cholesterol effusions. These effusions are also white or milky appearing but often occur in the presence of a trapped lung. A diagnosis of cholesterol effusion is made when the fluid cholesterol is greater than 200 mg/dL (5.18 mmol/L) and is confirmed by the presence of cholesterol crystals on microscopy.[8] Tuberculous empyema and rheumatoid pleurisy are the most common causes. Cholesterol accumulates from the breakdown of cellular membranes in these chronic effusions.

Yellow Nail Syndrome

Yellow nail syndrome (YNS) is a rare disorder characterized by the triad of classic-appearing thickened yellow nails (**Fig. 4**), lymphedema, and chronic respiratory complaints. It is included here because its cause is thought to be a functional disruption of lymphatic drainage, which would explain the formation of pleural effusions and lymphedema. Several entities have been associated but most are probably spurious.[9] Intestinal lymphangiectasia has been described in association with protein-losing enteropathy.

Pleural effusions occur in 40% of patients with YNS and are typically discordant exudates.[9] The protein is typically high but LDH low, as in chylous effusions. Chylous effusions compose 30% of the effusions in YNS. Treatment is often supportive but may include vitamin E for the yellow nails; compression stockings for lymphedema; and procedures beyond thoracentesis for pleural disease, including pleurodesis or thoracic duct ligation.[13,14]

Urinothorax

Urinothorax is defined by the presence of urine in the pleural space. It should be suspected during thoracentesis if the fluid has an odor and appearance of urine and should be considered in patients with a pleural effusion and obstructive uropathy.

Recent investigators have proposed dividing cases of urinothorax into 2 separate categories depending on the causative pathologic condition: obstructive urinothorax or traumatic urinothorax. Although urinary obstruction is fairly common in clinical practice, urinothorax is quite uncommon, with the literature being limited to case reports and small series. Obstruction can be related to nephrolithiasis; renal cysts, malignancy; retroperitoneal fibrosis; or congenital malformations, most commonly posterior urethral valves. Obstructive urinothorax is more commonly seen in bilateral ureteral or distal urinary tract obstruction and only rarely in unilateral ureteral obstruction if the contralateral kidney is functioning normally.[15] Traumatic urinothorax has been reported with cases of blunt abdominal trauma and iatrogenic injury. Implicated procedures include percutaneous nephrostomy tube placement, kidney biopsy, and various intraabdominal surgical procedures.[15] It is thought that disruption of the urinary tract leads to leakage of urine into the retroperitoneal space and formation of urinomas. Urine then enters the pleural space either through the lymphatic drainage or via direct defects in the diaphragm. Urinothorax is usually unilateral with fluid collecting ipsilateral to the side of injury, although there have been reported cases of collection on the contralateral side.[16] Although the cause of urinary injury may be known in many cases and seen via conventional imaging, there have been reports of occult fistulas. In these cases, renal scintigraphy with radioactive

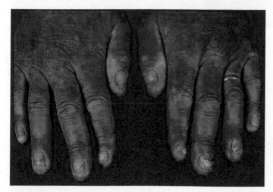

Fig. 4. The classic appearance of fingernails in YNS. (*From* Danielsson A, Toth E, Thorlacius H. Capsule endoscopy in the management of a patient with a rare syndrome–yellow nail syndrome with intestinal lymphangiectasia. Gut 2006;55(2):196, 233; with permission.)

tracer may allow the clinician to visualize the tract and confirm the diagnosis.[17]

Urinothorax is generally characterized by a transudative effusion with a low glucose and a low pH, although a high LDH has been reported.[15] The diagnosis is made by the measurement of the pleural fluid creatinine level. Stark and colleagues[18] suggested that a ratio of pleural fluid to serum creatinine greater than one is considered diagnostic. More recent investigators have demonstrated this ratio to be similarly elevated in other conditions; therefore, care must be taken to confirm the diagnosis.[15]

Pancreaticopleural Fistula

Pancreaticopleural fistula is defined by the communication between the pancreatic duct and pleural space, leading to the accumulation of pancreatic secretions in the pleural space. It is most commonly associated with chronic or recurrent pancreatitis,[19] although it can occur after an episode of acute pancreatitis or from iatrogenic causes (endoscopic retrograde cholangiopancreatography [ERCP]-induced pancreatitis, surgical pancreatectomy).[20] With each of these injuries, there is inflammation of the pancreatic duct, which can lead to stricture formation, ductal hypertension, and eventual disruption. Depending on the location of the injury, pancreatic fluid can either move anteriorly into the peritoneum, leading to pancreatic ascites, or posteriorly into the retroperitoneum, where it can migrate into the pleural space.[21]

Patients with pancreaticopleural fistula often present with dyspnea, chest or abdominal pain,

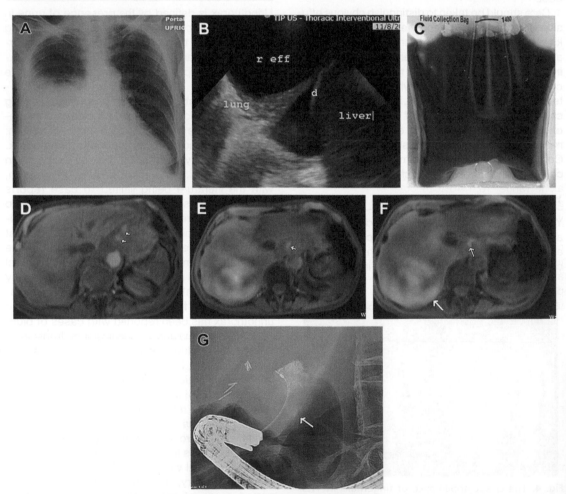

Fig. 5. (A) CXR demonstrating a large right pleural effusion. (B) Ultrasound confirmed the effusion and a thoracentesis was performed, with the fluid shown in (C). (D) After identifying an elevated amylase, MRCP showed a fistulous connection between a pancreatic pseudocyst and the right pleural space. (E, F) Serial images on MRCP with arrows pointing to the fistulous tract. (G) ERCP was subsequently performed with transpapillary placement of a stent into the pseudocyst to promote drainage away from the fistulous tract. CXR, Chest X-ray.

or cough.[22] After radiography demonstrates an effusion, pleural fluid analysis typically reveals a serosanguinous, exudative fluid with markedly elevated amylase levels.[23] The mean amylase value in one large series was 47 362 U/L (range 400–446 600 U/L). In contrast to patients with effusions related to acute pancreatitis who may also have elevated pleural fluid amylase, those with fistula formation are likely to have larger effusions, rapid reaccumulation of fluid after removal, and higher levels of pleural fluid amylase. Pleural fluid amylase values greater than 50 000 U/L seldom, if ever, occur in the absence of a fistula.[22,23]

The fistulous tract can often be identified by imaging. A large review demonstrated the sensitivity of computed tomography (47%) was less than that of magnetic resonance cholangiopancreatography (MRCP, 80%). ERCP had a sensitivity of 78% in the same review and has the added advantage of providing potential therapy.[22] **Fig. 5** gives a representative case of a pancreaticopleural fistula identified by MRCP and treated with ERCP.

Conservative management attempts to decrease pancreatic fluid production and treat symptoms, which is accomplished by either elemental enteral feeds or TPN. In addition to dietary changes, somatostatin (or its analogue octreotide) is thought to decrease pancreatic exocrine function and slow fluid production.[22] Some investigators advocate at least a 2- to 4-week conservative trial to facilitate closure.[23] Success rates for conservative therapy alone range from 40% to 65% in most reports, although the exact risk factors for failure have not yet been clearly identified.

Advances in ERCP techniques have dramatically changed the treatment of pancreaticopleural fistulas. ERCP can help identify the fistulous track and simultaneously enable stent placement in the pancreatic duct to bypass the pathology, leading to decreased output into the pleural space because the pancreatic duct is more patent. Some investigators have suggested that ERCP with stenting, along with octreotide, should be the first-line therapy in patients with significant strictures. In one case series of 11 patients successfully treated for pancreaticopleural fistulas, there were no symptomatic recurrences at more than 4 years of follow-up.[24] With the development of pancreatic stenting, the need for surgical intervention has been dramatically reduced and indicated only for patients that fail.

OTHER RARE SUBDIAPHRAGMATIC CAUSES OF PLEURAL EFFUSIONS

Other subdiaphragmatic structures may be associated with pleural effusions. Biliopleural fistulas have been reported after radiofrequency ablation for hepatocellular carcinoma,[25] transarterial chemoembolization of liver lesions,[26,27] and percutaneous transhepatic gallbladder drainage.[28] Other causes include infections (hydatid cyst) and trauma. Gastropleural fistulas have been associated with peptic ulcer disease, trauma, malignancy, surgery, and other causes. Duodenopleural and colopleural fistulas have been reported. A splenic echinococcal cyst burrowing into the left pleural space has also been described.[29] Thus, virtually any intra-abdominal organ may communicate in one way or another with the pleural space.

SUMMARY

In summary, intra-abdominal fluid may migrate readily into the pleural space through naturally occurring holes in the diaphragm or intradiaphragmatic lymphatics. Although any type of fluid in the abdomen may migrate, additional pathologic mechanisms are involved for the development of chylous ascites/chylothorax, YNS, urinothorax, pancreaticopleural fistulas, or other connections. In the differential diagnosis of the large list of potential pleural fluid causes, intra-abdominal sources should be entertained by the practicing physician in the right clinical context.

REFERENCES

1. Light RW. Pleural diseases. 4th edition. Baltimore: Lippincott, Williams & Wilkins; 2001.
2. Panicek DM, Benson CB, Gottlieb RH, et al. The diaphragm: anatomic, pathologic, and radiologic considerations. Radiographics 1988;8(3):385–425.
3. Abu-Hijleh MF, Habbal OA, Moqattash ST. The role of the diaphragm in lymphatic absorption from the peritoneal cavity. J Anat 1995;186(Pt 3): 453–67.
4. Hematti H, Mehran RJ. Anatomy of the thoracic duct. Thorac Surg Clin 2011;21(2):229–38, ix.
5. Kinasewitz GT, Keddissi JI. Hepatic hydrothorax. Curr Opin Pulm Med 2003;9(4):261–5.
6. Lepage S, Bisson G, Verreault J, et al. Massive hydrothorax complicating peritoneal dialysis. Isotopic investigation (peritoneopleural scintigraphy). Clin Nucl Med 1993;18(6):498–501.
7. Cheng MH, Yen MS, Chao KC, et al. Differential diagnosis of gynecologic organ-related diseases in women presenting with ascites. Taiwan J Obstet Gynecol 2008;47(4):384–90.
8. Huggins JT. Chylothorax and cholesterol pleural effusion. Semin Respir Crit Care Med 2010;31(6): 743–50.

9. Ryu JH, Tomassetti S, Maldonado F. Update on uncommon pleural effusions. Respirology 2011; 16(2):238–43.

10. Kalomenidis I. Octreotide and chylothorax. Curr Opin Pulm Med 2006;12(4):264–7.

11. Mares DC, Mathur PN. Medical thoracoscopic talc pleurodesis for chylothorax due to lymphoma: a case series. Chest 1998;114(3):731–5.

12. Zabeck H, Muley T, Dienemann H, et al. Management of chylothorax in adults: when is surgery indicated? Thorac Cardiovasc Surg 2011;59(4):243–6.

13. Maldonado F, Tazelaar HD, Wang CW, et al. Yellow nail syndrome: analysis of 41 consecutive patients. Chest 2008;134(2):375–81.

14. Maldonado F, Ryu JH. Yellow nail syndrome. Curr Opin Pulm Med 2009;15(4):371–5.

15. Garcia-Pachon E, Padilla-Navas I. Urinothorax: case report and review of the literature with emphasis on biochemical diagnosis. Respiration 2004;71(5):533–6.

16. Dimitriadis G, Tahmatzopoulos A, Kampantais S, et al. Unilateral urinothorax can occur contralateral to the affected kidney. Scand J Urol Nephrol 2012. [Epub ahead of print].

17. Jelic S, Sampogna RV. Detection of unrecognized urinothorax with renal scintigraphy. Kidney Int 2009;76(3):353.

18. Stark DD, Shanes JG, Baron RL, et al. Biochemical features of urinothorax. Arch Intern Med 1982; 142(8):1509–11.

19. Gomez-Cerezo J, Barbado CA, Suarez I, et al. Pancreatic ascites: study of therapeutic options by analysis of case reports and case series between the years 1975 and 2000. Am J Gastroenterol 2003;98(3):568–77.

20. Sut M, Gray R, Ramachandran M, et al. Pancreatico-pleural fistula: a rare complication of ERCP-induced pancreatitis. Ulster Med J 2009;78(3):185–6.

21. Eckhauser F, Raper SE, Knol JA, et al. Surgical management of pancreatic pseudocyst, pancreatic ascites, and pancreaticopleural fistulas. Pancreas 1991;6(Suppl 1):S66–75.

22. Ali T, Srinivasan N, Le V, et al. Pancreaticopleural fistula. Pancreas 2009;38(1):e26–31.

23. Rockey DC, Cello JP. Pancreaticopleural fistula. Report of 7 patients and review of the literature. Medicine (Baltimore) 1990;69(6):332–44.

24. Roberts KJ, Sheridan M, Morris-Stiff G, et al. Pancreaticopleural fistula: etiology, treatment and long-term follow-up. Hepatobiliary Pancreat Dis Int 2012;11(2):215–9.

25. Azcarate-Perea L, Moreno-Mata N, Gonzalez-Casaurran G, et al. Biliopleural fistula after radiofrequency ablation of hepatocellular carcinoma. Rev Esp Enferm Dig 2011;103(9):494–6.

26. Butt AS, Mujtaba G, Anand S, et al. Management of biliopleural fistula after transarterial chemoembolization of a liver lesion. Can J Gastroenterol 2010;24(5): 281–3.

27. Lewis JR, Te HS, Gehlbach B, et al. A case of biliopleural fistula in a patient with hepatocellular carcinoma. Nat Rev Gastroenterol Hepatol 2009;6(4):248–51.

28. Lee MT, Hsi SC, Hu P, et al. Biliopleural fistula: a rare complication of percutaneous transhepatic gallbladder drainage. World J Gastroenterol 2007; 13(23):3268–70.

29. Barzilai A, Pollack S, Kaftori JK, et al. Splenic echinococcal cyst burrowing into left pleural space. Chest 1977;72(4):543–5.

Treatment of Complicated Pleural Effusions in 2013

Rahul Bhatnagar, MB ChB, MRCP[a,b],
Nick A. Maskell, DM, FRCP[b,c],*

KEYWORDS

- Complicated pleural effusions • Pleural effusions • Pleural infections • Lung infections
- Fibrinolytic therapy • Empyema

KEY POINTS

- The treatment of complicated pleural effusions caused by infection continues to evolve.
- The worldwide incidence is increasing with a changing spectrum of causative organisms and underlying causes.
- Although often related to a pneumonic illness, there is little correlation between organisms typically found in the pleural space and those usually associated with parenchymal lung infections, suggesting primary pleural infection is far more common than previously believed, and that the term parapneumonic effusion is therefore often not an accurate label.
- Early recognition and instigation of simple therapies such as antibiotics, nutritional supplements, and chest drainage remain the cornerstone of good management.
- For an important subgroup of patients, fibrinolytic therapy seems to enable full recovery without surgical methods.
- Larger randomized trials are needed in this area to fully clarify their role, but recent evidence suggests that combination therapy with deoxyribonuclease (DNase) is likely to lead to the best outcomes for patients.

The word complicated, when used to describe a pleural effusion, can be applied in several contexts. The various descriptions encompass fluid collections that have begun to develop visible fibrin deposition, have become abnormally acidic, or require medical intervention to ensure resolution.[1] Although changes such as these may be caused by pleural malignancy, or even by some benign processes,[2] the term complicated pleural effusion has become synonymous with the commonest cause: pleural space infection.

The incidence of pleural infection seems to be increasing worldwide,[3–5] but despite continued advances in the management of this condition, morbidity and mortality have essentially remained static over the past decade. The quest for improvements in this field has resulted in an active international research community, which continues to

Funding Sources: Dr Bhatnagar has received lecture fees from AstraZeneca and GlaxoSmithKline, and educational grants from Novartis and GlaxoSmithKline. Dr Maskell has received research funding from Novartis and CareFusion. He has also received honoraria from CareFusion for medical advisory board meetings.
Conflicts of Interest: Dr Bhatnagar and Dr Maskell have no conflicts of interests to declare.
[a] Respiratory Research Unit, Southmead Hospital, Southmead Road, Westbury-on-Trym, Bristol BS10 5NB, UK;
[b] Academic Respiratory Unit, University of Bristol, Second Floor, Learning and Research, Southmead Hospital, Southmead Road, Westbury-on-Trym, Bristol BS10 5NB, UK; [c] North Bristol Lung Unit, Southmead Hospital, Southmead Road, Westbury-on-Trym, Bristol BS10 5NB, UK
* Corresponding author. North Bristol Lung Unit, Southmead Hospital, Southmead Road, Westbury-on-Trym, Bristol BS10 5NB, UK.
E-mail address: nick.maskell@bristol.ac.uk

chestmed.theclinics.com

work to further the understanding of the underlying pathophysiology. Beneficial effects on the provision of health care are also anticipated from new techniques for early detection and risk stratification.[3]

This article summarizes the current evidence and opinions on the epidemiology, etiology, and management of complicated pleural effusions caused by infection, including empyema. Although many parallels may be drawn between children and adults in such cases, most trials, guidelines, and series regard pediatric patient groups and those more than 18 years of age as separate entities.[6] This review focuses mainly on the treatment of adult disease.

HISTORICAL PERSPECTIVE

The first historical references to pleural infection have been credited to the ancient Egyptians, around 5000 years ago.[7] However, it was Hippocrates who first described empyema through his revolutionary bedside-based and dissection-based approach to medicine around 400 BC.[8] Medical practices were not significantly challenged again until the late nineteenth century when French physicians revisited the Hippocratic method with a modern eye.[9] Until this time, open thoracic drainage of empyema was the standard of care, however there was a 70% mortality rate with this treatment. Closed tube drainage was described but not adopted widely until the formation of an Empyema Commission shortly after World War I, when the ravages of the influenza pandemic and its inevitable pleural sequelae forced the introduction of significant management changes.[10] A landmark paper by Graham[11] charted the successes seen during this time, with short-term mortality plummeting to 3.4% in certain treatment camps. He went on to describe in great detail the etiology, physiology, microbiology, and outcomes of empyema thoracis and its treatment at the time, laying the foundation for modern approaches. The ensuing 90 years were punctuated by further significant advances in the management of pleural infection, although perhaps not to the degree that was hoped for.[12] Widespread availability of antibiotics, vaccination programs, and video-assisted surgery have had an impact on both microbiology and long-term morbidity, with further improvements hopefully still to be gained by the use of intrapleural fibrinolytic therapy.[6]

EPIDEMIOLOGY

Despite these advances, recent literature has shown that the incidence of infection-related complicated pleural effusion is increasing. This seems to be the case for both children and adults, and although most data are derived from populations in the developed world, this pattern has been replicated worldwide.[3,4,13–15] Between 20% and 57% of patients who develop pneumonia go on to develop a parapneumonic effusion,[16–18] and although most of these patients do not require invasive treatment or investigation, a small subgroup may experience serious complications. Of the approximately 1 million cases of hospitalized pneumonia each year in the United States, around 60,000 develop frank empyema. A further 25,000 are estimated to develop empyema for other reasons, including trauma and iatrogenic instrumentation.[1] These figures do not necessarily take into account effusions deemed complicated due to bacterial isolation or fibrous septations, which almost certainly makes the true burden of pleural infection much greater. Grijalva and colleagues[5] recently examined the trends in parapneumonic empyema in the United States over a 13-year period in a recent publication. This study relied heavily on disease coding practices in hospitals but was still able to demonstrate a doubling in the rate of hospitalization due to empyema between 1996 and 2008, from 3.04 to 5.98 per 100,000. Similar results were demonstrated by a Canadian study, which also confirmed the significant disparity in empyema incidence between those aged 65 years or more (17–20 per 100,000) and those aged 19 years or less (2–4 per 100,000).[3] Taking into account the average number of bed days for such patients, the average cost of managing patients with pleural infections in the United States and the United Kingdom probably exceeds $300 million per year.[19]

Mortality rates from empyema also seem to be on the increase. A study looking at the population of Utah showed a marked increase in mortality between 2000 and 2005 compared with the relatively stable rates between 1950 and 1999.[20] Absolute percentage mortality was low (<4%) in this group, but figures from other series have recorded mortality among standard inpatients up to 18% in the short-term,[21] with those in intensive care experiencing mortality as high as 41%.[22] In a large multicenter trial from the United Kingdom, in which the average patient age was 59 years, the 1-year mortality rate after treatment for empyema ranged between 8% and 20%.[19]

MICROBIOLOGY

Understanding of pleural infection microbiology has traditionally involved extrapolation from the organisms implicated in pneumonia. Theoretic evidence supports this, at least in part, as exemplified in a recent study by Wilkosz and colleagues[23] who demonstrated a murine model for the transfer of upper airway bacterial isolates into the pleural space. Although there are undoubtedly patients who experience something similar, mounting evidence suggests that the bacteriology of pleural infection, and perhaps the condition itself, should be considered as a distinct entity.[24] The infected pleural space has significant differences in acidity and oxygenation compared with aerated lung, lending itself to invasion by certain organisms more than others.[25] Furthermore, there is incomplete radiographic correlation between pneumonia and pleural infection, and an inability for many traditional pneumonia severity scores to accurately predict the outcome of pleural infection.[26] Similar differences exist between pleural infections acquired in the community and those acquired in health care settings; the latter group is occasionally further subdivided into those who have iatrogenic intervention and those who have passive exposure to infection.

The first major shift in the type of bacteria causing pleural infection occurred after the introduction of antibiotics. Before this, around two-thirds of community-acquired cases were attributable to

Streptococcus pneumonia; this figure subsequently dropping to around 10%.[27] Precise definition of the cause is challenging, however. Ex vivo culture is difficult, particularly with the early and aggressive use of antibiotics, which can mask bacterial isolates.[28] The highest yield using standard culture techniques seems to be around 60%, with the inoculation of standard blood culture bottles the most convenient method for achieving this.[29,30] A large study of patients in the United Kingdom with pleural infection (**Fig. 1**) combined standard methods with nucleic acid amplification to discern causative organisms; a 74% overall identification rate was attained. Cloning techniques were also applied to a small number of cases (3%), limited by cost. DNA studies were able to identify an organism in 38% of the culture-negative samples; the same organism was found by both culture and nucleic acid amplification (or cloning) in 35% of cases. Of these, culture was only able to provide more complete information about the organism 6% of the time and DNA studies 8% of the time. A technique was deemed superior when it was able to find an organism not picked up by the other. Using this rule, culture was better in 26% of cases and nucleic acid amplification in 13% of cases. In 12%

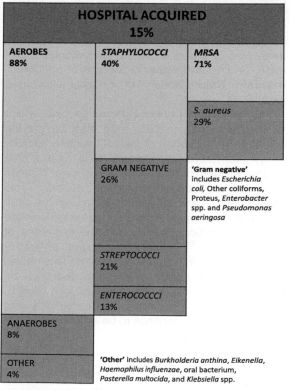

Fig. 1. Description of the bacteriology of pleural infection. Figures are derived from the total number of bacterial isolates achieved using standard culture and DNA amplification techniques (n = 336 for community-acquired, n = 60 for hospital-acquired). Of 434 individual cases analyzed, 88 (20%) were polymicrobial.

of cases there was conflicting information from the tests and so a clear assessment could not be made.

In this cohort, the *Streptococcus anginosus* group (formerly *S milleri* group) was the predominant set of bacteria. These and other gram-positive aerobes were implicated in 65% of cases, confirming the inherent differences in etiology compared with pneumonia. Other organisms included *Staphylococci* (11%), gram-negative aerobes such as *Escherichia coli* (9%), and anaerobes (20%).[31] Polymicrobial samples were identified in 20% of cases, but this may well underestimate the true incidence, as suggested by the cloning techniques used in the study and the fact that anaerobes have been identified in up to three-quarters of cases of community-acquired pleural infection in other series.[32]

Hospital-acquired pleural infection made up only 15% of the UK cohort, but the differences between these cases and community-acquired cases was marked. Most (58%) cases were attributed to gram-negative organisms or *Staphylococci*; more than 70% of the latter were caused by methicillin-resistant *Staphylococcus aureus* (MRSA).[31] Similar gram-negative predominance has been found among patients admitted to the intensive care setting.[22] These findings have led to a shift in the antibiotics suggested for empirical treatment of pleural infections, and to the development of specific guidelines for their management.[6] Although necessarily region specific, the recommendations acknowledge the likelihood of *Streptococcal* and anaerobic coinfection in community-acquired disease, and for the higher proportion of multidrug-resistant *Staphylococci* in hospital-associated disease.[31]

The heptavalent pneumococcal vaccine, which was introduced in 2000, may also be playing a role in the evolution of pleural infection bacteriology. Numerous investigators have noted a shift in the predominant serotypes causing disease toward those not covered by the vaccine.[33] This phenomenon has been described in both the adult and pediatric populations, and seems to correlate with the significant increase in the incidence of empyema,[13,14,34] suggesting a degree of heightened virulence in the new organisms. This makes it all the more important that the approach to, and understanding of, complicated pleural effusions is based on current evidence, and that descriptive series continue to be attempted alongside the interventional.

PATHOGENESIS AND TERMINOLOGY

As alluded to earlier, confusion may occasionally arise from the terms used to describe the processes and conditions involved in pleural infection. The phrase complicated pleural effusion and the word empyema are sometimes used interchangeably, and although convenient, this approach presupposes the lack of disease spectrum and potential significant clinical differences between patients. A useful clinical classification describes infection-related effusions as being complicated when invasive or semi-invasive intervention becomes necessary because of the presence of bacteria in the fluid, or when biochemical markers within it suggest the development of significant inflammation. The term empyema should be used based on visual appearances, with the presence of pus in the chest as its defining feature.[1] This typically represents a later, and often more therapeutically challenging, degree of pleural involvement.

The processes that lead to pneumonia-associated empyema are typically broken down into 3 phases (**Fig. 2**), with the transition between them varying greatly from one patient to the next. The trigger is usually the aspiration of oropharyngeal bacteria and the development of pneumonic changes over approximately 1 week. Primary pleural infection, without pneumonia, probably arises as a result of hematogenous spread from similar areas.[35] An uncomplicated effusion may develop over the next few days, representing an exudative stage, which becomes complicated during the subsequent fibrinopurulent stage. An empyema forms during the longer-lasting organizational stage, reflected in the indolent clinical course in some of those affected. The overall timeframe for the development of empyema can depend on several factors, including the patient's own immunity and the virulence of the infecting organism. This means that, although some patients may progress rapidly, it is also not unusual to find others deteriorating over 4 to 6 weeks.[1]

Initial pleural fluid formation is usually a direct consequence of localized inflammation and immune system activation. The processes involved may be likened to those involved in wound healing and begin with increased capillary vascular permeability as a result of endothelial injury caused by activated neutrophils, which form the bulk of the immune cells in early complicated effusions.[36,37] This allows fluid to move into the pleural space, which in normal circumstances contains around 10 mL of liquid,[38] with the resulting accumulation caused by an imbalance in the ratio of production to lymphatic drainage. At this stage, pleural fluid sampling reveals an exudative effusion, but does not demonstrate significant acidity (pH is >7.2), a notable decrease in glucose, or an increase in lactate dehydrogenase (LDH).[2]

Ongoing pleural insult leads to the development of the fibrinopurulent phase, with activation of

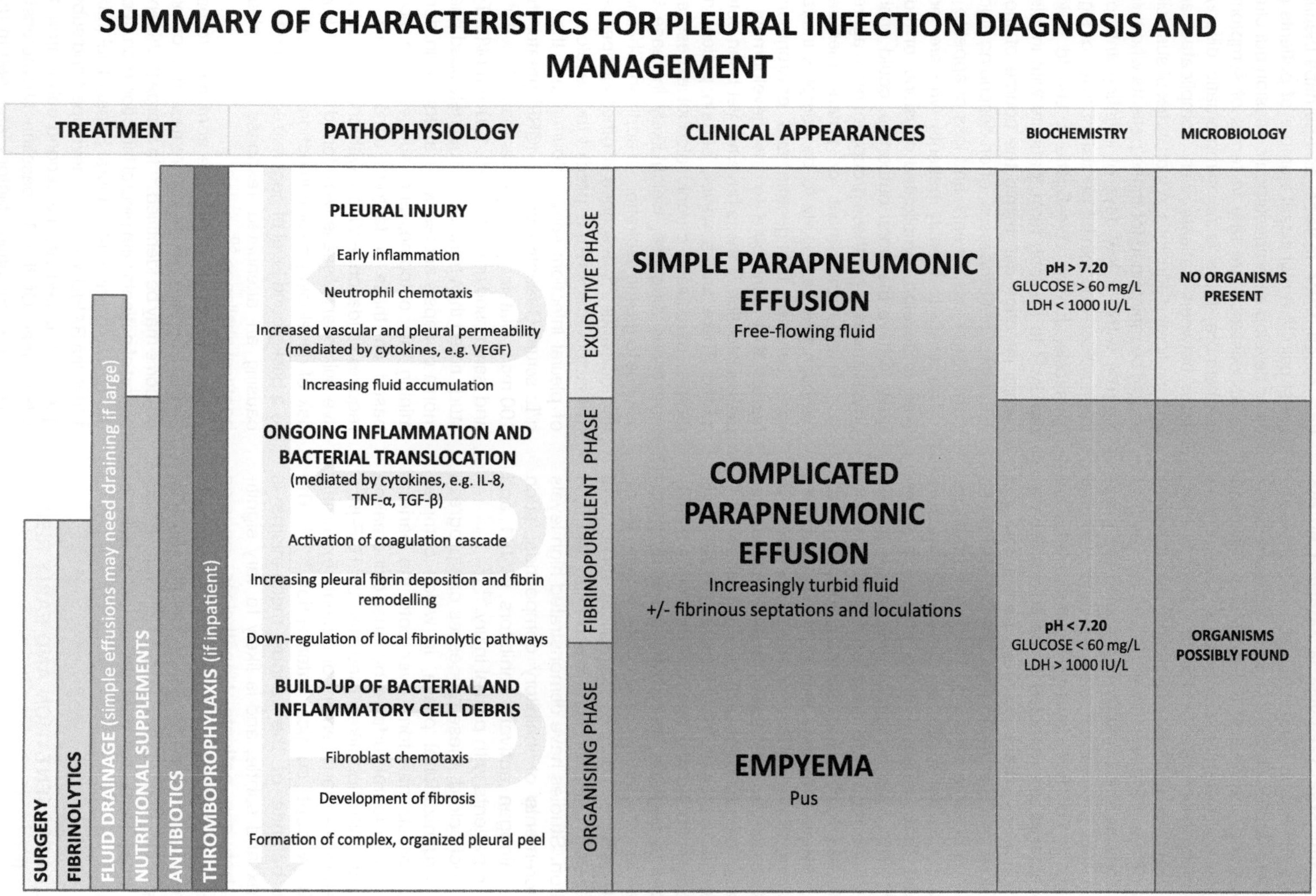

SUMMARY OF CHARACTERISTICS FOR PLEURAL INFECTION DIAGNOSIS AND MANAGEMENT

TREATMENT	PATHOPHYSIOLOGY		CLINICAL APPEARANCES	BIOCHEMISTRY	MICROBIOLOGY

PATHOPHYSIOLOGY

PLEURAL INJURY

Early inflammation

Neutrophil chemotaxis

Increased vascular and pleural permeability (mediated by cytokines, e.g. VEGF)

Increasing fluid accumulation

ONGOING INFLAMMATION AND BACTERIAL TRANSLOCATION
(mediated by cytokines, e.g. IL-8, TNF-α, TGF-β)

Activation of coagulation cascade

Increasing pleural fibrin deposition and fibrin remodelling

Down-regulation of local fibrinolytic pathways

BUILD-UP OF BACTERIAL AND INFLAMMATORY CELL DEBRIS

Fibroblast chemotaxis

Development of fibrosis

Formation of complex, organized pleural peel

PHASES: EXUDATIVE PHASE · FIBRINOPURULENT PHASE · ORGANISING PHASE

CLINICAL APPEARANCES

SIMPLE PARAPNEUMONIC EFFUSION
Free-flowing fluid

COMPLICATED PARAPNEUMONIC EFFUSION
Increasingly turbid fluid
+/- fibrinous septations and loculations

EMPYEMA
Pus

BIOCHEMISTRY

pH > 7.20
GLUCOSE > 60 mg/L
LDH < 1000 IU/L

pH < 7.20
GLUCOSE < 60 mg/L
LDH > 1000 IU/L

MICROBIOLOGY

NO ORGANISMS PRESENT

ORGANISMS POSSIBLY FOUND

TREATMENT

THROMBOPROPHYLAXIS (if inpatient)

ANTIBIOTICS

NUTRITIONAL SUPPLEMENTS

FLUID DRAINAGE (simple effusions may need draining if large)

FIBRINOLYTICS

SURGERY

Fig. 2. The pathophysiology, appearance, diagnostic parameters, and treatment options of infected pleural effusions.

proinflammatory and profibrotic components, as well as initiation of the coagulation cascade. The local inflammatory response is amplified by the presence of various cytokines, such as transforming growth factor (TGF)-β, tumor necrosis factor (TNF)-α, and interleukin (IL)-8, which stimulate neutrophil and fibroblast chemotaxis.[37] Membrane permeability makes recordable bacterial translocation most likely during this period, and the later stages of this process can lead to the expected visual appearance of empyema due to the presence of cell breakdown products and bacterial remnants.[39] The high level of cellular respiration and lactic acid are reflected in the fluid biochemistry, which by definition now has a low pH (<7.2), low glucose level, and LDH level 3 times normal.[2] A notable exception to this are effusions caused by *Proteus* species, which can secrete enzymes that cause a more alkaline environment.[40] The overall intrapleural effect of the cellular infiltration is to downregulate fibrinolysis, thus increasing fibrin formation using locally available substrate. A major component in this process is plasminogen, which can normally be cleaved to the active compound plasmin by enzymes such as urokinase plasminogen activator or tissue plasminogen activator (t-PA).[41] This forms the basis for modern fibrinolytic therapy. Plasmin normally functions to degrade fibrin clots, and so its inhibition can lead to many of the changes seen in the pleural space during complicated pleural processes, typified by fibrous septation and fluid loculation. Studies have demonstrated high levels and increments of inhibitory compounds, such as plasminogen activator inhibitors (PAI)-1 and PAI-2, in patients with pleural injury.[41,42]

Left unchecked, these processes can progress to the organizational phase, in which complex pleural fibrosis can form over both the parietal and visceral pleural surfaces because of increased fibroblast infiltration (likely mediated by TGF-β[43]), and can make management of patients extremely difficult without surgical intervention.[44–46] The overall balance of the various mechanisms is complex and subtle, and is likely to vary significantly between patients. Nonetheless, ongoing clarification of these processes continues, with the ultimate aim of being able to identify sensitive and specific biomarkers, and to provide efficacious treatments to patients at all stages of disease.

CLINICAL PRESENTATION AND EARLY RISK STRATIFICATION

Although there have been some extremely unusual cases,[47] the classic presentation of prolonged pleural infection is difficult to separate from that of pneumonia, whereby patients suffer with dyspnea, cough, fever, malaise, and perhaps pleuritic chest pain.[18] A significant number of patients go on to develop a parapneumonic effusion but clues to its existence are rare in terms of symptoms. Furthermore, there is no symptomatic discriminator between patients with complicated and uncomplicated effusions. A high index of suspicion should be maintained for those patients who fail to improve within a few days of initiating antibiotic therapy[48] or who exhibit persistent fever or signs of sepsis; further investigations should follow rapidly.[49] In the long term, patients with indolent pleural infection can mimic the course of those with malignant processes, often describing significant weight loss, sweats, and loss of appetite.

The ability to identify patients who are most likely to develop complicated effusions, or those likely to have the worst outcomes, could enable physicians to target these groups for more aggressive initial management or potent therapies. Although there are likely to be complex interactions between the genetic and environmental factors that contribute to the development of pleural infection,[12] these have not yet been determined. There are, however, certain patient risk factors, particularly chronic alcohol excess and intravenous drug use, which likely increase the risk due to gastric aspiration. In addition, Chalmers and colleagues[26] described 4 other independent risk factors that seem to predict the development of pleural infection: serum albumin less than 30 g/L; serum C-reactive protein (CRP) greater than 100 mg/L; platelet count greater than 400×10^9/L; and serum sodium less than 130 mmol/L. This study noted than none of the routinely used pneumonia or sepsis scores were adequate in determining this outcome, and suggested a score based on these 6 factors, although this still requires validation. Patients with chronic obstructive pulmonary disease were found to be at lower risk of developing pleural infection, perhaps due to a background level of generalized inflammation causing an attenuated response to a pleural bacterial challenge.[50]

For those patients who are confirmed to have pleural infection, those at greatest risk of poor outcome may be identified.[51] In a large multicenter cohort of patients with pleural infection recruited to the UK Multicenter Intrapleural Sepsis Trial (MIST) 1 trial, the RAPID score was developed and subsequently validated using a second cohort from the MIST2 trial. Of the 32 baseline characteristics analyzed, 5 presenting factors (age, serum urea, serum albumin, fluid purulence, and likely origin of infection) could predict the eventual outcome, with patients divided into low-risk, medium-risk, or high-risk groups based on a score out of 7. Patients in the lowest risk group were found to have a mortality rate of less than 5% at 3 months, whereas those in the highest were found to have a mortality rate approaching 50% over the same period. The main potential advantage of this stratification system is that it allows physicians to institute fibrinolytics or surgery earlier in the clinical presentation when they are perhaps more likely to be successful.

IMAGING TECHNIQUE FOR PLEURAL INFECTION

Radiological tests form the cornerstone for the initial diagnosis and management of complicated pleural effusion. Radiographs, computed tomography (CT), ultrasonography (US), and other tools can detail the size, extent, nature, and potentially the cause of pleural effusions before any other intervention is undertaken. The standard chest radiograph is a valuable screening tool because of its ubiquity and low radiation dose. Fluid collections greater than 250 mL are usually appreciable although the cause of the fluid may not be apparent. The suspicion of a complicated pleural process should be raised if the lung seems to be indented by pleural shadowing in way that is not consistent with the expected effects of gravity on fluid (**Fig. 3**).[52]

CT and US have become part of the standard approach to many pleural conditions. The use of US enables a radiation-free bedside assessment of fluid echogenicity, an approximation of volume, and can guide thoracentesis or chest tube placement. The degree of septation and loculation can be better appreciated than on CT scans (**Fig. 4**), allowing a strong inference of the presence of a complicated effusion or empyema in the right clinical setting.[53] US can also be used to improve the safety and accuracy of pleural sampling and drain insertion,[54,55] because images are viewed in real time.

Imaging of the pleura is best undertaken using CT. In addition, the ability to reconstruct images allows for a greater appreciation of the overall fluid burden as well as potential parenchymal causes such as pneumonia or obstructing lesions.[56] By obtaining images approximately 20 to 60 seconds after contrast administration, with slices of 1 to 3 mm, a clear delineation between lung and pleural tissue can usually be made, especially if the lung is atelectatic.[57] Features suggestive of pleural infection include the presence of air in the pleural space (in the absence of recent instrumentation) (**Fig. 5**) and smooth pleural thickening that spares the mediastinal surfaces. In cases of empyema or otherwise infected pleural fluid, the split pleura sign can often be appreciated due to visceral and parietal pleural enhancement surrounding a fluid collection (**Fig. 6**), occasionally in conjunction with increased attenuation of extrapleural fat.[58] Despite a strong case for their regular use in the assessment of pleural infection, and despite some physicians' tendencies,[59] currently neither CT nor US can reliably predict the outcome of an effusion after chest tube insertion or fibrinolytic therapy,[60] nor which patients should be selected for a particular surgical intervention.[61]

As a result of the accuracy achieved by these imaging modalities, the role for others, such as magnetic resonance imaging (MRI) and positron emission tomography (PET), is restricted. MRI is capable of similar diagnostic accuracy to CT scans but the images are easily degraded by

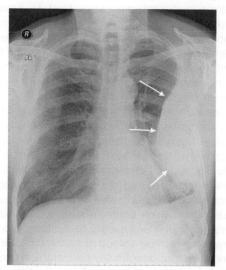

Fig. 3. Chest radiograph showing a loculated pleural effusion. Note how the pleural shadow (*outlined by arrows*) does not conform to the expected effects of gravity on fluid, suggesting a more complicated process.

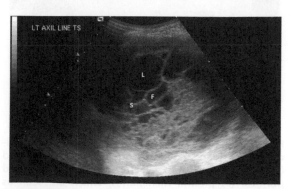

Fig. 4. Thoracic ultrasound scan showing multiple septations (S), loculation (L), and echogenic fluid (F).

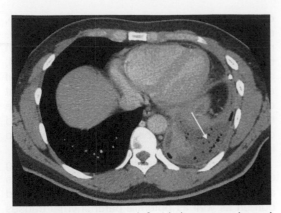

Fig. 5. CT scan showing a left-sided empyema (*arrow*). Note how the fluid (*darker gray*) contains numerous bubbles (*black*), indicating the presence of gas-forming organisms. The fact that the bubbles have not coalesced suggests significant loculation, but this is not easily visualized using this modality.

respiratory motion and the scan is often more challenging for patients. Nonetheless, MRI may find use if spinal or rib involvement is suspected due to the infective process.[53] PET scanning in pleural infection is usually limited to when other modalities or tests have been unable to distinguish infection from pleural malignancy, because, although subtle, contrast uptake between these 2 conditions can differ.[62]

PLEURAL FLUID INVESTIGATION

Concerning signs, symptoms, or blood tests in the context of a suggestive radiograph should lead to confirmation of effusion and early fluid sampling. However, in a small retrospective series by Skouras

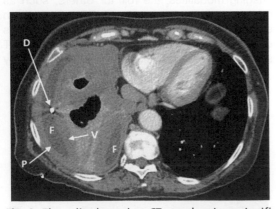

Fig. 6. The split pleura sign. CT scan showing a significant right-sided empyema. Note how the pleural fluid (F) is outlined by markedly thickened visceral (V) and parietal (P) pleural membranes, which are seen as a result of a delayed contrast scan protocol. A chest drain (D) is in situ.

and colleagues,[63] the investigators suggested that parapneumonic effusions less than 2 cm in depth on US can be treated without further sampling as they are unlikely to become complicated or require intervention. Even if confirmed in larger prospective studies, such patients require close monitoring and appropriate antibiotic therapy.

Once the effusion has been sampled, routine tests should include fluid pH, protein, LDH, and glucose. Increased levels of cellular respiration and breakdown within the fluid cause dynamic changes in these values, with the development of a complex parapneumonic effusion suggested by the presence of a pH value less than 7.2, an LDH level greater than 1000 IU/L, and a glucose level less than 60 mg/dL (3.4 mmol/L).[6] As described earlier, the yield from sending a sample for Gram stain and bacterial culture may be significantly improved by inoculating a blood culture bottle with a few milliliters of the initial aspirate.[29] If there is a suspicion of mycobacterial involvement, adenosine deaminase levels along with stain and culture for acid-fast bacilli may be of diagnostic use; extended viral or fungal studies may also be useful in patients who are significantly immunocompromised. In addition, because repeated thoracentesis is itself a risk-factor for pleural infection, and because there are occasions when primarily malignant effusions can mimic complicated infective effusions, recommendations state that fluid be sent for cytologic examination along with these other baseline tests.[64] The discovery of a neutrophil-predominant or macrophage-predominant effusion may guide management toward that of infection, whereas malignant processes tend to produce lymphocytic exudates.[65] A degree of diagnostic caution should always be maintained, however, as inflammatory effusions are likely to transition from being neutrophil-predominant or macrophage-predominant to lymphocyte-predominant if present for more than 2 weeks.

The best solitary discriminator for a complicated pleural process during initial investigations is fluid pH level. Many studies demonstrate better patient outcomes when drainage is instituted based on the early biochemical changes related to infection.[66] Current guidelines regard a pH of 7.2 as diagnostic of complexity, making this the definitive cutoff value below which drainage should take place.[6] Samples for pH can typically be processed within a few minutes using a blood gas analyzer, although samples that appear frankly purulent need not be tested for pH in this way because the visual appearance of empyema should prompt intervention irrespective of acidity.[1] Fluid pH values may be appreciably altered by minor variations in sampling and processing techniques, which can therefore have significant effects on management strategy. A study by Rahman and colleagues[67] reproduced several common scenarios that may occur during the testing of pleural fluid, and were able to demonstrate that even small amounts of residual heparin or local anesthetic in a sample syringe can dramatically lower pH results. The opposite was found when residual air was left in the syringe; pH increased by an average of 0.08 if 2 mL of fluid was exposed to 1 mL of air. This represented a clinically significant change in more than two-thirds of patients.

ADDITIONAL FLUID INVESTIGATIONS

Glucose, LDH, and pH measurements determine whether an effusion is complicated and have been shown to be extremely sensitive discriminators. However, a retrospective analysis by Porcel and colleagues[68] showed that these tests were not particularly specific when it came to establishing the need for chest tube drainage in nonpurulent effusions, meaning a subset of patients may undergo unnecessary treatments. Other fluid biomarkers have been investigated to help guide diagnostics and therapeutic interventions.

In recent years, many potential markers have been tested focusing on different parts of the inflammatory and infective cascades. These include complement products (C5b-9)[69]; enzymes (myeloperoxidase)[70]; acute phase reactants (CRP and procalcitonin)[71–73]; markers of oxidative stress[74]; and cytokines (TNF-α and IL-8).[75,76] It has also been suggested that the absolute neutrophil count in fluid can be useful.[77] Both pleural fluid CRP and vascular endothelial growth factor have been suggested as long-term predictors for developing residual pleural thickening.[78,79] Although the sensitivity and specificity of some of these tests can be extremely good,[36] none have so far been proved to be superior in differentiating between uncomplicated and complicated effusions compared with the existing methods. Further clarification and experimentation is needed before any new marker can be adopted, although skepticism exists on whether the ideal biomarker will ever be found.[12]

BASIC THERAPIES
Antibiotics and Chest Drainage

The need for supportive and preventative care is great in those with pleural infection, as many are toward the severe end of the sepsis spectrum and will perhaps be more immobile after intervention. Early institution of thromboembolic prophylaxis is recommended for most medical inpatients,[80] and the use of calorie supplements should not be

delayed if needed, remembering that empyema is more common in groups who are predisposed to nutritional impairment. As discussed earlier, the empirical use of antibiotics or other antimicrobials should be based on local guidelines and patient-specific risks. Patients often show signs of generalized sepsis at presentation, and systemic antibiotics are frequently administered before pleural fluid cultures can be taken or analyzed. Previous studies have shown that the concentrations of parenterally administered penicillins and cephalosporins within a parapneumonic effusion are up to 75% of those found in serum,[81] and similarly high pleural levels of metronidazole were found in an animal model of empyema.[82] These antibiotics allow a broad spectrum of coverage, including anaerobes. Alternative antibiotic classes and agents that have shown good pleural penetrance, albeit rarely in true clinical scenarios, are carbapenems, ciprofloxacin, clindamycin, and chloramphenicol.[6] Because of these results, little work has been done to explore intrapleural antibiotic instillation despite it being intuitively appealing, especially as little is known about antibiotic levels in fluid surrounded by thickened pleura. There is also limited understanding regarding the activity of such antibiotics in highly acidic environments, circumstances that may explain why studies have shown aminoglycoside levels to be undetectable in empyema when given intravenously.[83,84]

Historically, patients suspected of having pleural infection had larger chest drains inserted. Although never formally proved, this recommendation was largely based on the fear of small tubes becoming blocked with the viscous fibrous products likely to be drained in these situations. However, current practice has begun to shift toward the use of smaller drains because evidence of their noninferiority has begun to mount. A large Taiwanese series used small (10–16 French) pigtail catheters to manage a range of pleural conditions. Most of these were used for cases of pleural infection, with a reported success rate of 72%.[85] A retrospective analysis of the large MIST1 cohort demonstrated no significant difference in the rates of surgical referral or mortality depending on drain size.[86] This same analysis showed patients with larger drains were more likely to suffer pain from their tube, although there may have been bias introduced because the drain size was not randomized (drain size was determined by local physicians, meaning those with empyema, and perhaps more inflamed pleura, may have received larger drains).[87]

The lack of formal randomized studies means that there is as yet no formal consensus on the issue of optimal drain size, but the latest British

Thoracic Society guidelines now suggest 10 to 14 French chest tubes can be used first line in cases of complicated pleural effusion.[6] These drains can usually be inserted safely using the Seldinger technique and are best managed after insertion with regular sterile flushes to ensure drain patency. Some European centers use regular saline irrigation to manage complex effusions with the aim of removing pleural debris in conjunction with systemic therapy. Such a concept is plausible, even if the only studies thus far relate to postoperative infected pleural collections; these studies have also tested the idea of pleural sterilization using antibiotic irrigation.[88]

Fibrinolytic Therapy

Early knowledge of the fibrotic processes underlying complicated pleural effusions led to the first use of intrapleural streptokinase more than 60 years ago.[89] However, it is only in the last 10 to 15 years that significant advances have been made in determining the most appropriate role for this class of medication in pleural infection; more work is still needed.

Davies and colleagues[90] were able to begin to allay long-standing safety fears regarding intrapleural thrombolysis in a small series of 24 patients; improvements in clinical outcomes were also noted in those given streptokinase. Other studies tended to focus more on the use of urokinase in loculated effusions; benefits were demonstrated in terms of treatment failure (as judged by surgical referral or death), surgical outcome, and length of hospital stay.[91–93] However, these studies tended to be small trials or case series, which limited their generalizability.

The MIST1 trial[94] recruited 454 patients with pleural infection from around the United Kingdom to receive either streptokinase or placebo. Entry criteria reflected real-world practice with a strong reliance on diagnosis by a local physician, antibiotic choice, chest tube use, and surgical referral. The trial was unable to show any significant benefit from the use of streptokinase in either levels of surgical referral or death, and was supported by a subsequent meta-analysis. However, a Cochrane review found that intrapleural fibrinolytics conferred benefit in both treatment failure and the need for surgical intervention in loculated effusions or empyema, but not mortality.[95] Criticism of the MIST1 trial largely stemmed from its design. The use of small-bore chest tubes was questioned, as was the inclusion of patients who did not have loculated effusions, and because centralized drug distribution may have led to treatment delays.[90,96] The choice of streptokinase as the primary lytic

may also have contributed to these results, because its mechanism of action relies on using a proportion of the intrapleural plasminogen to form an active complex before the rest can be converted to plasmin.[97] Nonetheless, the 2010 British Thoracic Guidelines went on to state that intrapleural fibrinolytics should not be used routinely, but may be considered in select cases.[6]

The MIST2 trial was published in 2011 by Rahman and colleagues.[19] It hypothesized that the addition of intrapleural deoxyribonuclease (DNase) to standard fibrinolytic therapy (recombinant t-PA) would confer extra benefit in the treatment of empyema and complicated pleural effusions. This hypothesis was based on previous observations that similar combinations in animal models had resulted in reduced empyema viscosity, presumably through the supplemental breakdown of DNA-based debris within the fluid.[98] Recruitment took place over 3 years from 11 UK centers and patients were selected on clinical criteria. A higher proportion (91.4%) of patients had loculated effusions at baseline compared with those in MIST1. The primary end point was change in radiographic pleural opacification and patients were randomized to receive 1 of 4 treatments: double placebo, DNase plus placebo alone, t-PA plus placebo, or t-PA plus DNase. Although the actual numbers of patients receiving each treatment were small, those who received DNase and t-PA in combination were found to have significantly improved radiographic outcomes, lower rates of surgical referral at 3 months, and a mean hospital stay of almost a week less than those receiving placebo alone. The finding that isolated treatment with either of the study drugs produced results similar to placebo potentially supports the findings of the earlier MIST trial, and led the investigators to suggest that future studies should be directed toward larger-scale combination trials. This sentiment was echoed in a 2012 meta-analysis that included the results of this study. They reported similar findings to the previous Cochrane review, noting significant heterogeneity in study results, but suggesting potential benefits by reducing treatment failure with antifibrin treatment.[99] A summary of the double-blind placebo-controlled trials that have looked at fibrinolytic therapy is shown in **Fig. 7**.

As the documented evolution of the use of thrombolytic therapy demonstrates, there is undoubtedly a great deal left to discover regarding their true role in the management of complicated pleural effusions. Work continues to try and refine thrombolytic molecules, with a plasmin-activated urokinase precursor demonstrating, in animal models, reduced susceptibility to PAI-1 inhibition, increased

SUMMARY OF DOUBLE-BLIND, PLACEBO-CONTROLLED TRIALS OF FIBRINOLYTIC THERAPY

STUDY	STUDY SIZE	INCLUSION	DRAIN SIZE	TREATMENT	MORTALITY (%) treatment	MORTALITY (%) placebo	SURGICAL REFERRAL RATE (%) treatment	SURGICAL REFERRAL RATE (%) placebo
Davies et al [90] 1997	24	Empyema and complex effusions	14 Fr	Streptokinase Once daily Three days	0	0	0	25
Bouros et al [91] 1999	31	Empyema and complex effusions	28-32 Fr	Urokinase Once daily Three days	0	0	13	38
					Not significant		P<.05	
Tuncozgur et al [92] 2001	49	Empyema only	24-36 Fr	Urokinase Once daily Three days	0	0	29	60
					Not significant		P<.001	
Diacon el al [93] 2004	53	Empyema and complex effusions	24-28 Fr	Streptokinase Once daily Seven days	4.5	4.5	14	45.5
					Not significant		P = .02	
Maskell et al [94] MIST1 2005	454	Empyema and complex effusions	12-20 Fr	Streptokinase Twice daily Three days	15.5	14	15.5	14.5
					Not significant		Not significant	
Rahman et al [19] MIST2 2011	210	Empyema and complex effusions	<15 Fr	t-PA and DNAse Twice daily Three days	8	4	4	16
					Not significant		P = .03	
					NO OVERALL DIFFERENCE		FIBRINOLYTICS FAVORED OVERALL [99]	

Fig. 7. Summary of double-blind placebo-controlled trials of fibrinolytic therapy.

fibrin selectivity, and a half-life that would potentially allow for single-dose administration.[37]

Surgical Options

Referral for surgical intervention usually occurs after failed medical treatment (antibiotics, chest drain insertion, and fibrinolytics), or with late presentations with highly organized empyemas showing marked pleural fibrosis. Practice tends to vary, but some centers have an extremely low threshold for early surgery, especially as the overall costs can be comparable with medical treatments.[100] The point at which medical management is deemed to have failed is necessarily ill-defined; the risks of a particular surgical procedure are highly dependent on individual patient factors. Surgical involvement should be considered with significant loculation, which may predispose to long-term respiratory impairment, and/or ongoing signs of sepsis despite adequate antibiotic therapy.

Surgical options are varied and may be tailored to the individual. Video-assisted thoracoscopic surgery (VATS) typically requires general anesthetic and single-lung ventilation, but these requirements can be relaxed in the face of significant comorbidities. Although originally used for thorough pleural debridement,[101] VATS can now be used to perform decortication in particularly advanced or chronic empyema, although the latter situation may reduce the chance of a successful outcome.[102] Despite this, the overall success rate for VATS exceed 85%.

Open decortication for empyema was formerly a mainstay of treatment, but as evidence has emerged to show that VATS is at least comparable, and perhaps even superior,[103] its role is likely to become increasingly marginalized, being used only when the less invasive approach has failed. Decortication after thoracotomy allows complete mobilization of the lung, which is particularly useful in cases of trapped lung.[104] It may ensure that maximum symptomatic benefit is gained from 1 operation, although this may be at the expense of a more prolonged recovery. A study from 1996 described a mortality rate of about 3% for this operation.[105]

For patients who have recurrent or particularly complex empyema, small prosthetic devices may be inserted between ribs to maintain a permanent drainage route. The more extreme way to achieve this effect is to perform an open-window thoracostomy. This procedure involves the resection of 2 or 3 ribs to create a direct opening to the thoracic cavity, which affords the opportunity to pack the pleural space at the expense of creating an aesthetic alteration to the chest wall.[106] Should methods such

as these fail, a thoracomyoplasty may become necessary, whereby a large muscle is used to pack the thoracic cavity. This procedure is usually reserved for patients with bronchopleural fistulae, trapped lung, or postoperative empyema.[104]

SUMMARY

The treatment of complicated pleural effusions caused by infection continues to evolve. The worldwide incidence is increasing with a changing spectrum of causative organisms and underlying causes. Although often related to a pneumonic illness, there is little correlation between organisms typically found in the pleural space and those usually associated with parenchymal lung infections, suggesting primary pleural infection is far more common than previously believed, and that the term parapneumonic effusion is therefore often not an accurate label. Thus, there is an ever-growing appreciation of the complex processes involved and pleural infection is increasingly being recognized as an entirely separate entity. Specialized tools have now been developed and validate to allow physicians to more accurately predict the likely progress of patients and the potential to target treatment.

Early recognition and instigation of simple therapies such as antibiotics, nutritional supplements, and chest drainage remains the cornerstone of good management. However, for an important subgroup of patients, fibrinolytic therapy seems to enable full recovery without surgical methods. Larger randomized trials are needed in this area to fully clarify their role, but recent evidence suggests that combination therapy with DNase is likely to lead to the best outcomes for patients.

REFERENCES

1. Sahn SA. Diagnosis and management of parapneumonic effusions and empyema. Clin Infect Dis 2007;45(11):1480–6.
2. Light RW. Parapneumonic effusions and empyema. Proc Am Thorac Soc 2006;3(1):75–80.
3. Finley C, Clifton J, Fitzgerald JM, et al. Empyema: an increasing concern in Canada. Can Respir J 2008;15(4):219.
4. Farjah F, Symons RG, Krishnadasan B, et al. Management of pleural space infections: a population-based analysis. J Thorac Cardiovasc Surg 2007;133(2):346–51.
5. Grijalva CG, Zhu Y, Nuorti JP, et al. Emergence of parapneumonic empyema in the USA. Thorax 2011;66(8):663–8.
6. Davies HE, Davies RJ, Davies CW. Management of pleural infection in adults: British Thoracic Society

Pleural Disease Guideline 2010. Thorax 2010; 65(Suppl 2):ii41–53.

7. Breasted J. The Edwin Smith surgical papyrus. Chicago: University of Chicago Press; 1980.

8. Hippocrates. Section 5(8). Aphorisms. Available at: http://classics.mit.edu/Hippocrates/aphorisms.5.v.html Accessed November 28, 2012.

9. Bynum W. The history of medicine: a very short introduction. Oxford (United kingdom): Oxford University Press; 2008.

10. Peters RM. Empyema thoracis: historical perspective. Ann Thorac Surg 1989;48(2):306–8.

11. Graham E. Some fundamental considerations in the treatment of empyema thoracis. St Louis (MO): CV Mosby; 1925.

12. Tobin CL, Lee YC. Pleural infection: what we need to know but don't. Curr Opin Pulm Med 2012; 18(4):321–5.

13. Masson A, Menetrey C, Garnier F, et al. Parapneumonic pleural effusion incidence in a French region before and during the antipneumococcal vaccine era. Arch Pediatr 2011;18(8):846–9.

14. Goldbart AD, Leibovitz E, Porat N, et al. Complicated community acquired pneumonia in children prior to the introduction of the pneumococcal conjugated vaccine. Scand J Infect Dis 2009; 41(3):182–7.

15. Wu PS, Huang LM, Chang IS, et al. The epidemiology of hospitalized children with pneumococcal/lobar pneumonia and empyema from 1997 to 2004 in Taiwan. Eur J Pediatr 2010; 169(7):861–6.

16. Taryle DA, Potts DE, Sahn SA. The incidence and clinical correlates of parapneumonic effusions in pneumococcal pneumonia. Chest 1978;74(2):170–3.

17. Bartlett JG, Finegold SM. Anaerobic infections of the lung and pleural space. Am Rev Respir Dis 1974;110(1):56–77.

18. Light RW, Girard WM, Jenkinson SG, et al. Parapneumonic effusions. Am J Med 1980;69(4):507–12.

19. Rahman NM, Maskell NA, West A, et al. Intrapleural use of tissue plasminogen activator and DNase in pleural infection. N Engl J Med 2011; 365(6):518–26.

20. Bender JM, Ampofo K, Sheng X, et al. Parapneumonic empyema deaths during past century, Utah. Emerg Infect Dis 2009;15(1):44–8.

21. Ferguson AD, Prescott RJ, Selkon JB, et al. The clinical course and management of thoracic empyema. QJM 1996;89(4):285–9.

22. Tu CY, Hsu WH, Hsia TC, et al. The changing pathogens of complicated parapneumonic effusions or empyemas in a medical intensive care unit. Intensive Care Med 2006;32(4):570–6.

23. Wilkosz S, Edwards LA, Bielsa S, et al. Characterization of a new mouse model of empyema and the mechanisms of pleural invasion by Streptococcus pneumoniae. Am J Respir Cell Mol Biol 2012;46(2): 180–7.

24. Marrie TJ, editor. Community acquired pneumonia. New York: Plenum Press; 2001.

25. Whiley RA, Beighton D, Winstanley TG, et al. Streptococcus intermedius, Streptococcus constellatus, and Streptococcus anginosus (the Streptococcus milleri group): association with different body sites and clinical infections. J Clin Microbiol 1992;30(1): 243–4.

26. Chalmers JD, Singanayagam A, Murray MP, et al. Risk factors for complicated parapneumonic effusion and empyema on presentation to hospital with community-acquired pneumonia. Thorax 2009;64(7):592–7.

27. Heffner JE. Diagnosis and management of thoracic empyemas. Curr Opin Pulm Med 1996; 2(3):198–205.

28. Becker A, Amantea SL, Fraga JC, et al. Impact of antibiotic therapy on laboratory analysis of parapneumonic pleural fluid in children. J Pediatr Surg 2011;46(3):452–7.

29. Menzies SM, Rahman NM, Wrightson JM, et al. Blood culture bottle culture of pleural fluid in pleural infection. Thorax 2011;66(8):658–62.

30. Ferrer A, Osset J, Alegre J, et al. Prospective clinical and microbiological study of pleural effusions. Eur J Clin Microbiol Infect Dis 1999;18(4):237–41.

31. Maskell NA, Batt S, Hedley EL, et al. The bacteriology of pleural infection by genetic and standard methods and its mortality significance. Am J Respir Crit Care Med 2006;174(7):817–23.

32. Bartlett JG, Thadepalli H, Gorbach SL, et al. Bacteriology of empyema. Lancet 1974;303(7853):338–40.

33. Lisboa T, Waterer GW, Lee YC. Pleural infection: changing bacteriology and its implications. Respirology 2011;16(4):598–603.

34. Hendrickson DJ, Blumberg DA, Joad JP, et al. Five-fold increase in pediatric parapneumonic empyema since introduction of pneumococcal conjugate vaccine. Pediatr Infect Dis J 2008; 27(11):1030–2.

35. Koegelenberg CF, Diacon AH, Bolliger CT. Parapneumonic pleural effusion and empyema. Respiration 2008;75(3):241–50.

36. Porcel JM. Pleural fluid tests to identify complicated parapneumonic effusions. Curr Opin Pulm Med 2010;16(4):357–61.

37. Idell S. The pathogenesis of pleural space loculation and fibrosis. Curr Opin Pulm Med 2008;14(4): 310–5.

38. Noppen M, De Waele M, Li R, et al. Volume and cellular content of normal pleural fluid in humans examined by pleural lavage. Am J Respir Crit Care Med 2000;162(3 Pt 1):1023–6.

39. Kroegel C, Antony VB. Immunobiology of pleural inflammation: potential implications for pathogenesis,

diagnosis and therapy. Eur Respir J 1997;10(10): 2411–8.

40. Pine JR, Hollman JL. Elevated pleural fluid pH in *Proteus mirabilis* empyema. Chest 1983;84(1): 109–11.

41. Idell S, Girard W, Koenig KB, et al. Abnormalities of pathways of fibrin turnover in the human pleural space. Am Rev Respir Dis 1991;144(1):187–94.

42. Philip-Joët F, Alessi MC, Philip-Joët C, et al. Fibrinolytic and inflammatory processes in pleural effusions. Eur Respir J 1995;8(8):1352–6.

43. Vassalli JD, Sappino AP, Belin D. The plasminogen activator/plasmin system. J Clin Invest 1991;88(4): 1067–72.

44. Idell S, Pendurthi U, Pueblitz S, et al. Tissue factor pathway inhibitor in tetracycline-induced pleuritis in rabbits. Thromb Haemost 1998;79(3):649–55.

45. Idell S, Mazar A, Cines D, et al. Single-chain urokinase alone or complexed to its receptor in tetracycline-induced pleuritis in rabbits. Am J Respir Crit Care Med 2002;166(7):920–6.

46. Strange C, Baumann MH, Sahn SA, et al. Effects of intrapleural heparin or urokinase on the extent of tetracycline-induced pleural disease. Am J Respir Crit Care Med 1995;151(2 Pt 1):508–15.

47. Sharma JK, Marrie TJ. Explosive pleuritis. Can J Infect Dis 2001;12(2):104–7.

48. Lim WS, Baudouin SV, George RC, et al. BTS guidelines for the management of community acquired pneumonia in adults: update 2009. Thorax 2009;64(Suppl 3):iii1–55.

49. Sahn SA, Light RW. The sun should never set on a parapneumonic effusion. Chest 1989;95(5):945–7.

50. Torres A, Menéndez R. Mortality in COPD patients with community-acquired pneumonia: who is the third partner? Eur Respir J 2006;28(2):262–3.

51. Maskell NA, Kahan BC, Rahman NM. Rapid score – the first validated clinical score in pleural infection to identify those at risk of poor. Am J Respir Crit Care Med 2012;185:A5431.

52. de Lacey G, Morley S, Berman L. The chest X-ray: a survival guide. Philadelphia: Saunders Elsevier; 2008.

53. Heffner JE, Klein JS, Hampson C. Diagnostic utility and clinical application of imaging for pleural space infections. Chest 2010;137(2):467–79.

54. Lamont T, Surkitt-Parr M, Scarpello J, et al. Insertion of chest drains: summary of a safety report from the National Patient Safety Agency. BMJ 2009;339:b4923.

55. Diacon AH, Brutsche MH, Solèr M. Accuracy of pleural puncture sites: a prospective comparison of clinical examination with ultrasound. Chest 2003;123(2):436–41.

56. Ravenel JG, McAdams HP. Multiplanar and three-dimensional imaging of the thorax. Radiol Clin North Am 2003;41(3):475–89.

57. Evans AL, Gleeson FV. Radiology in pleural disease: state of the art. Respirology 2004;9(3):300–12.

58. Aquino SL, Webb WR, Gushiken BJ. Pleural exudates and transudates: diagnosis with contrast-enhanced CT. Radiology 1994;192(3):803–8.

59. Chen KY, Liaw YS, Wang HC, et al. Sonographic septation: a useful prognostic indicator of acute thoracic empyema. J Ultrasound Med 2000; 19(12):837–43.

60. Gervais DA, Levis DA, Hahn PF, et al. Adjunctive intrapleural tissue plasminogen activator administered via chest tubes placed with imaging guidance: effectiveness and risk for hemorrhage. Radiology 2008;246(3):956–63.

61. Roberts JR. Minimally invasive surgery in the treatment of empyema: intraoperative decision making. Ann Thorac Surg 2003;76(1):225–30 [discussion: 229–30].

62. Toaff JS, Metser U, Gottfried M, et al. Differentiation between malignant and benign pleural effusion in patients with extra-pleural primary malignancies: assessment with positron emission tomography-computed tomography. Invest Radiol 2005;40(4): 204–9.

63. Skouras V, Awdankiewicz A, Light RW. What size parapneumonic effusions should be sampled? Thorax 2010;65(1):91.

64. Hooper C, Lee YC, Maskell N. Investigation of a unilateral pleural effusion in adults: British Thoracic Society Pleural Disease Guideline 2010. Thorax 2010;65(Suppl 2):ii4–17.

65. Porcel JM. Pearls and myths in pleural fluid analysis. Respirology 2011;16(1):44–52.

66. Heffner JE, Brown K, Barbieri C, et al. Clinical commentary pleural fluid chemical analysis in parapneumonic effusions. Am J Respir Crit Care Med 1995;151(6):1700–8.

67. Rahman NM, Mishra EK, Davies HE, et al. Clinically important factors influencing the diagnostic measurement of pleural fluid pH and glucose. Am J Respir Crit Care Med 2008;178(5):483–90.

68. Manuel Porcel J, Vives M, Esquerda A, et al. Usefulness of the British Thoracic Society and the American College of Chest Physicians guidelines in predicting pleural drainage of non-purulent parapneumonic effusions. Respir Med 2006;100(5):933–7.

69. Vives M, Porcel JM, Gázquez I, et al. Pleural SC5b-9: a test for identifying complicated parapneumonic effusions. Respiration 2000;67(4):433–8.

70. Alegre J, Jufresa J, Segura R, et al. Pleural-fluid myeloperoxidase in complicated and noncomplicated parapneumonic pleural effusions. Eur Respir J 2002;19(2):320–5.

71. Lin MC, Chen YC, Wu JT, et al. Diagnostic and prognostic values of pleural fluid procalcitonin in parapneumonic pleural effusions. Chest 2009; 136(1):205–11.

72. San Jose ME, Valdes L, Vizcaino LH, et al. Procalcitonin, C-reactive protein, and cell counts in the diagnosis of parapneumonic pleural effusions. J Investig Med 2010;58(8):971–6.

73. Porcel JM, Vives M, Cao G, et al. Biomarkers of infection for the differential diagnosis of pleural effusions. Eur Respir J 2009;34(6):1383–9.

74. Tsilioni I, Kostikas K, Kalomenidis I, et al. Diagnostic accuracy of biomarkers of oxidative stress in parapneumonic pleural effusions. Eur J Clin Invest 2011;41(4):349–56.

75. Porcel JM, Vives M, Esquerda A. Tumor necrosis factor-alpha in pleural fluid: a marker of complicated parapneumonic effusions. Chest 2004; 125(1):160–4.

76. Porcel JM, Galindo C, Esquerda A, et al. Pleural fluid interleukin-8 and C-reactive protein for discriminating complicated non-purulent from uncomplicated parapneumonic effusions. Respirology 2008;13(1):58–62.

77. San Jose ME, Valdes L, Gonzalez-Barcala FJ, et al. Diagnostic value of proinflammatory interleukins in parapneumonic effusions. Am J Clin Pathol 2010; 133(6):884–91.

78. Skouras V, Boultadakis E, Nikoulis D, et al. Prognostic value of C-reactive protein in parapneumonic effusions. Respirology 2012;17(2):308–14.

79. Papaioannou AI, Kostikas K, Tsopa P, et al. Residual pleural thickening is related to vascular endothelial growth factor levels in parapneumonic pleural effusions. Respiration 2010;80(6):472–9.

80. Hill J, Treasure T. Reducing the risk of venous thromboembolism in patients admitted to hospital: summary of NICE guidance. BMJ 2010;340:c95.

81. Taryle DA, Good JT, Morgan EJ, et al. Antibiotic concentrations in human parapneumonic effusions. J Antimicrob Chemother 1981;7(2):171–7.

82. Teixeira LR, Sasse SA, Villarino MA, et al. Antibiotic levels in empyemic pleural fluid. Chest 2000; 117(6):1734–9.

83. Thys JP, Vanderhoeft P, Herchuelz A, et al. Penetration of aminoglycosides in uninfected pleural exudates and in pleural empyemas. Chest 1988; 93(3):530–2.

84. Shohet I, Yellin A, Meyerovitch J, et al. Pharmacokinetics and therapeutic efficacy of gentamicin in an experimental pleural empyema rabbit model. Antimicrob Agents Chemother 1987;31(7):982–5.

85. Liu YH, Lin YC, Liang SJ, et al. Ultrasound-guided pigtail catheters for drainage of various pleural diseases. Am J Emerg Med 2010;28(8):915–21.

86. Rahman NM, Maskell NA, Davies CW, et al. The relationship between chest tube size and clinical outcome in pleural infection. Chest 2010;137(3):536–43.

87. Light RW. Pleural controversy: optimal chest tube size for drainage. Respirology 2011;16(2):244–8.

88. Ng T, Ryder BA, Maziak DE, et al. Treatment of postpneumonectomy empyema with debridement followed by continuous antibiotic irrigation. J Am Coll Surg 2008;206(3):1178–83.

89. Sherry S, Johnson A, Tillett WS. The action of streptococcal desoxyribose nuclease (streptodornase) in vitro and on purulent pleural exudations of patients. J Clin Invest 1949;28(5 Pt 2): 1094–104.

90. Davies RJ, Traill ZC, Gleeson FV. Randomised controlled trial of intrapleural streptokinase in community acquired pleural infection. Thorax 1997;52(5):416–21.

91. Bouros D, Schiza S, Tzanakis N, et al. Intrapleural urokinase versus normal saline in the treatment of complicated parapneumonic effusions and empyema. A randomized, double-blind study. Am J Respir Crit Care Med 1999;159(1):37–42.

92. Tuncozgur B, Ustunsoy H, Sivrikoz MC, et al. Intrapleural urokinase in the management of parapneumonic empyema: a randomised controlled trial. Int J Clin Pract 2001;55(10):658–60.

93. Diacon AH, Koegelenberg CF, Bolliger CT. A trial of intrapleural streptokinase. N Engl J Med 2005; 352(21):2243–5 [author reply: 2243–5].

94. Maskell NA, Davies CW, Nunn AJ, et al. UK controlled trial of intrapleural streptokinase for pleural infection. N Engl J Med 2005;352(9): 865–74.

95. Cameron R, Davies HR. Intra-pleural fibrinolytic therapy versus conservative management in the treatment of adult parapneumonic effusions and empyema. Cochrane Database Syst Rev 2008;(2):CD002312.

96. Heffner JE. Multicenter trials of treatment for empyema — after all these years. N Engl J Med 2005;352(9):926–8.

97. Young KC, Shi GY, Wu DH, et al. Plasminogen activation by streptokinase via a unique mechanism. J Biol Chem 1998;273(5):3110–6.

98. Zhu Z, Hawthorne ML, Guo Y, et al. Tissue plasminogen activator combined with human recombinant deoxyribonuclease is effective therapy for empyema in a rabbit model. Chest 2006;129(6): 1577–83.

99. Janda S, Swiston J. Intra-pleural fibrinolytic therapy for treatment of adult parapneumonic effusions and empyemas: a systematic review and meta-analysis. Chest 2012;142:401–11.

100. Shah SS, Ten Have TR, Metlay JP. Costs of treating children with complicated pneumonia: a comparison of primary video-assisted thoracoscopic surgery and chest tube placement. Pediatr Pulmonol 2010;45(1):71–7.

101. Yamaguchi M, Takeo S, Suemitsu R, et al. Video-assisted thoracic surgery for fibropurulent thoracic empyema: a bridge to open thoracic

surgery. Ann Thorac Cardiovasc Surg 2009; 15(6):368–72.

102. Luh SP, Chou MC, Wang LS, et al. Video-assisted thoracoscopic surgery in the treatment of complicated parapneumonic effusions or empyemas: outcome of 234 patients. Chest 2005;127(4):1427–32.

103. Chambers A, Routledge T, Dunning J, et al. Is video-assisted thoracoscopic surgical decortication superior to open surgery in the management of adults with primary empyema? Interact Cardiovasc Thorac Surg 2010;11(2):171–7.

104. Molnar TF. Current surgical treatment of thoracic empyema in adults. Eur J Cardiothorac Surg 2007;32(3):422–30.

105. Angelillo Mackinlay TA, Lyons GA, Chimondeguy DJ, et al. VATS debridement versus thoracotomy in the treatment of loculated postpneumonia empyema. Ann Thorac Surg 1996;61(6):1626–30.

106. Zahid I, Nagendran M, Routledge T, et al. Comparison of video-assisted thoracoscopic surgery and open surgery in the management of primary empyema. Curr Opin Pulm Med 2011;17(4):255–9.

Straightening Out Chest Tubes
What Size, What Type, and When

Kamran Mahmood, MD, MPH*,
Momen M. Wahidi, MD, MBA

KEYWORDS

- Chest tube • Tube thoracostomy • Small-bore chest tube • Large-bore chest tube • Pneumothorax
- Pleural effusion • Empyema • Hemothorax

KEY POINTS

- Although chest tubes range in size (6–40 French [Fr]) and shape (straight tubes vs pigtail catheters), small-bore tubes (<14 Fr) are effective for most pleural processes.
- Various types of pneumothorax and malignant and infected complicated pleural effusions have been successfully managed with small-bore chest tubes. Benefits of the smaller size include patient comfort and ease of placement.
- Large-bore chest tubes may be necessary for barotrauma-associated pneumothoraces in mechanically ventilated patients and in the postoperative setting. However, abundant literature supports a paradigm shift towards the more routine use of small-bore chest tubes for managing pleural disease.
- The Seldinger technique can be used for placement of small and large-bore chest tubes and ultrasound guidance is recommended.

Chest tube placement is one of the most common procedures performed to manage pleural disorders. The main purpose of tube thoracostomy is evacuation of air or fluid from the pleural cavity. Hippocrates first described its use in the fifth century BC for the treatment of empyema.[1] In 1876, Hewett[2] described the use of a bottle as a closed chest tube drainage system for management of empyema. Since then, chest tube design, methods of insertion, and drainage systems have evolved significantly.

Although chest tube placement is straightforward, it may be associated with significant morbidity and mortality. According to the United Kingdom National Patient Safety Agency, 12 deaths and 15 cases of serious harm occurred from chest tube placement in the United Kingdom between 2005 and 2008.[3] A survey of the hospitals in the United Kingdom also found a very high complication rate from chest tube placement, and stressed the importance of informed consent and proper training.[4] Thus, a need exists for enhancing the knowledge of various types of chest tubes and their placement techniques.

GUIDING CHEST TUBE PLACEMENT

Chest tubes are hollow cylindrical plastic catheters with drainage side holes designed for placement within the pleural cavity. Usually a radiopaque strip is present on the side of the chest tube to assist in visualization on chest radiographs. The most proximal hole of the chest tube, sentinel eye, is usually situated on this strip and visible on the chest radiograph as a defect in the line; this helps ensure that all drainage holes are inside the pleural cavity. Length markings on the tube note the distance of the sentinel eye from the skin insertion site.

Conflicts of Interest: None.
Division of Pulmonary, Allergy and Critical Care Medicine, Department of Medicine, Duke University Medical Center, DUMC 102356, Durham, NC 27710, USA
* Corresponding author.
E-mail address: k.mahmood@duke.edu

Clin Chest Med 34 (2013) 63–71
http://dx.doi.org/10.1016/j.ccm.2012.11.007

chestmed.theclinics.com

Chest tubes should be inserted into the "triangle of safety,"[3] an area bordered anteriorly by the lateral border of the pectoralis major, posteriorly by the lateral border of the latissimus dorsi, and inferiorly by a horizontal line at the level of the fifth intercostal space (**Fig. 1**). Staying in this triangle prevents injury to underlying vessels and organs. The chest tubes may be directed differently depending on the pathologic process. For pneumothorax, the tube is often aimed anterior and apical; for drainage of fluid, it is often directed posterior and basilar. For loculated effusions, the chest tube placement may be dictated by the location of the fluid.

Although various methods are used to correctly position chest tubes, including physical examination, fluoroscopy, and computed tomography (CT) scan, ultrasound is becoming increasingly popular to ensure proper placement. Ultrasound improves successful placement of the chest tube, especially in loculated pockets of pleural fluid.[5–7] Based largely on extrapolation of data from thoracentesis literature, ultrasound is believed to decrease the risk of chest tube misplacement or injury to surrounding organs.[8–12] The British Thoracic Society (BTS) pleural disease guidelines strongly recommend the use of ultrasound guidance for chest tube placement.[3]

CHEST TUBE TYPES BASED ON INSERTION TECHNIQUE

Chest tubes can be classified based on their method of insertion (**Table 1**), including blunt dissection into the pleura (**Fig. 2**), the Seldinger guidewire technique (**Figs. 3** and **4**), and the trocar

Table 1	
Chest tube methods of insertion and size	
Chest tube insertion methods	Blunt dissection Seldinger technique Placement by trocar
Chest tube sizes	Small-bore chest tube ($\leq$14 French) Large-bore chest tube (>14 French)

technique (**Fig. 5**). For various reasons, including a trend towards the use of smaller chest tubes and because of increased patient comfort, the Seldinger technique is becoming more popular in many institutions.

Blunt Dissection

Blunt dissection is the oldest technique for chest tube insertion. Using sterile technique and local anesthesia, an incision is made in the skin and subcutaneous tissue, parallel to the rib. The subcutaneous tissue and intercostal muscles are dissected and the pleural space is entered above the rib with the help of a clamp. Digital palpation of the pleural space is often performed and then the distal end of the chest tube is grasped with the clamp and directed into the pleural space.[3] The main advantages of this method include the ability to perform digital exploration in the pleural space, assessing for loculations and proper positioning, and the ability to direct the tube into the most appropriate position within the thoracic cavity. However, compared with the other techniques, this method is more painful, requires

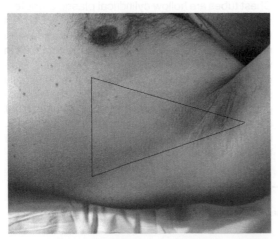

Fig. 1. Triangle of safety bordered by the pectoralis major, the latissimus dorsi, and a line at the level of the fifth intercostal space.

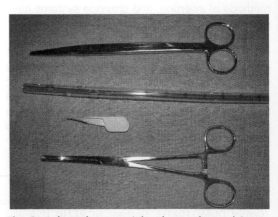

Fig. 2. A large-bore straight chest tube and instruments used for placement by blunt dissection (36-French, Argyle Straight Thoracic Catheter, Covidien, Mansfield, MA, USA; scissors; scalpel; forceps).

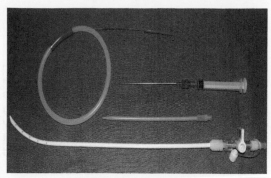

Fig. 3. A small-bore pigtail chest tube, commonly placed using the Seldinger technique (14-French, Wayne Pneumothorax Set, Cook Medical Inc, Bloomington, IN, USA; Guidewire; needle; dilator; chest tube).

a larger incision, and leaves a bigger scar after the tube is removed.

Seldinger Technique

Chest tubes placed by the Seldinger technique are placed with the help of a guidewire, and conceptually entail a similar process as central venous line placement. While using sterile technique and topical anesthesia, a needle is inserted into the pleural space with aspiration of fluid or air into a syringe. Thereafter, the guidewire is advanced through the needle, which is subsequently removed. One or more dilators are placed over the guidewire and advanced until a sensation of "give way" is felt on entry into the pleural space. The dilator is then removed and the chest tube, which is loaded on a stylet, is passed over the wire into the pleural space. On entering the pleural space, the chest tube is advanced into the pleural

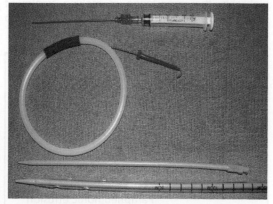

Fig. 4. A large-bore straight chest tube placed using the Seldinger technique (24-French, Thal-Quick Chest Tube, Cook Medical Inc, Bloomington, IN, USA; Needle; guidewire; dilator; chest tube).

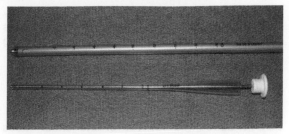

Fig. 5. Trocar straight chest tubes (24-French and 10-French, Argyle Trocar Catheter, Covidien, Mansfield, MA, USA). Note the sharp metal tip at the insertion ends.

space, the stylet is removed, and the tube is secured and attached to a drainage apparatus.[3] This technique may be used for both small and large chest tubes. The main advantages of this technique include the smaller incision, minimal tissue dissection resulting in less pain for the patient, and a more aesthetic scar after removal of the tube. Disadvantages include an inability to digitally manipulate the pleural space and limited ability to direct the tube to an exact location in the pleural space.

Trocar Placement

In this technique, a sharp-tipped rod (the trocar) is passed through the chest tube and then used to pierce the pleural space. An incision is made in the skin and subcutaneous tissue and the trocar/tube combination is pushed into the pleural space. The chest tube is left in the pleural space and the trocar withdrawn. Although technically simple, this "harpoon" technique has a high risk of complications, mainly because of the danger of impaling the lung or surrounding organs.[3,13–15] Hence, in the authors' opinion, these tubes are not recommended for routine use.

CHEST TUBE SIZE AND CONFIGURATION

Chest tubes come in a variety of sizes based on the external diameter, ranging from 6 to 40 French (Fr). One French is equal to one-third millimeter, and thus a 9-Fr chest tube is 3 mm in diameter. Broadly speaking, chest tubes may be straight or coiled at the end ("pig-tail"). Tunneled pleural catheters, discussed elsewhere in this issue by Myers and Michaud, are chest tubes used for out-patient long term management of pleural effusions and are tunneled to prevent dislodgement and infection. In the context of nonmalignant pleural disease, chest tubes are typically placed for hours or days. By convention, as shown in **Table 1**, a small-bore chest tube (SBCT) is typically 14 Fr or smaller, whereas a large-bore chest tube (LBCT) is typically more than 14 Fr in diameter. SBCTs are typically placed using the Seldinger technique, whereas LBCTs can be placed with dissection or using the Seldinger technique or a trocar.

ADVANTAGES AND DISADVANTAGES OF SMALL-BORE CHEST TUBES

SBCTs accounted for 7% of the chest tubes placed at a university health care system in the early 1990s.[16] However, the use of SBCTs is currently increasing.[17] Because of the smaller size, less to no dissection is required, and thus insertion tends to be less painful. Furthermore, the small incision usually causes less scar formation and typically does not require suturing after removal of the chest tube. Disadvantages of small-bore catheters include their lower flow rate, and thus the potential inability to evacuate large air leaks or rapid accumulation of viscous fluid, such as blood. An in vitro study comparing chest tubes of various sizes and manufacturers concluded that small-bore tubes have a significantly lower flow rate compared with the large-bore catheters.[18] Caution is advised to select a larger tube when big air leaks are expected, such as in patients on mechanical ventilation and with postpneumonectomy stump dehiscence. Finally, the flow of similar-sized tubes varies among different manufacturers, probably because of tube length and the material used to construct the catheter. Therefore, practitioners should be familiar with the chest tubes available in their institution before attempting chest tube placement.

Complications of SBCTs include injury to surrounding organs (0.2%), malposition (0.6%), empyema (0.2%), and drain blockage (8.1%).[3] Viscous fluids like blood or pus may clog the smaller chest tubes because of the low flow. The use of 30 mL of sterile saline to flush the tube every 6 to 8 hours can generally prevent tube blockage, and therefore routine flushing is advised.[19]

ADVANTAGES AND DISADVANTAGES OF LARGE-BORE CHEST TUBES

LBCTs have been conventionally placed for various reasons, including in the surgical field in the setting of trauma, postoperatively, and for empyema. LBCTs are less susceptible to clogging or kinking and are well suited for these indications. Disadvantages, however, include the need for tissue dissection, painful insertion, larger incisions, and a generally more invasive approach. Complications include injury to surrounding organs (1.4%), malposition (6.5%), empyema (1.4%), and drain blockage (5.2%).[3]

SMALL-BORE CHEST TUBES VERSUS LARGE-BORE CHEST TUBES IN DIFFERENT CLINICAL SCENARIOS

Several indications exist for chest tube placement (**Table 2**). This discussion summarizes the data surrounding the use of SBCTs versus LBCTs in these indications. The most challenging decision confronting physicians is most likely related to size of tube rather than whether it should be a straight or "pigtail" catheter and more studies are needed in this area.

Pneumothorax

Although LBCTs were initially thought necessary for patients with pneumothorax, several studies have shown the efficacy of smaller tubes for this indication. Because a pneumothorax may be large or small, iatrogenic or spontaneous, related or unrelated to underlying parenchymal disease, and have other variables, it is prudent to evaluate each type of pneumothorax individually when deciding the appropriate size of chest tube.

Primary spontaneous pneumothorax
It is important to determine if a spontaneous pneumothorax is primary or secondary. According to the recent BTS guidelines,[20] needle aspiration can be attempted as first-line management of primary spontaneous pneumothorax in patients if the pneumothorax is larger than 2 cm from the lung margin to the inside of the chest wall at the level of the hilum, as determined by chest radiograph, or if the patient is symptomatic. If simple aspiration fails to reexpand the lung, an SBCT should be inserted; LBCTs are not recommended. The American College of Chest Physicians defines a small pneumothorax as 3 cm or smaller, from the apex of the lung to the cupola.[21] This discrepancy highlights the importance of making treatment decisions based on patient symptoms while also

Table 2 Indications for tube thoracostomy	
Pneumothorax	Primary spontaneous pneumothorax Secondary spontaneous pneumothorax Traumatic pneumothorax Iatrogenic pneumothorax
Pleural effusions	Malignant pleural effusion Parapneumonic effusion and empyema Hemothorax Postoperative effusion

considering the size of the pneumothorax. CT scan of chest is more sensitive for evaluating the size of a pneumothorax.[20]

Multiple studies show that there is no significant difference in failure rate between LBCTs and SBCTs for primary spontaneous pneumothorax, thus supporting the role of the small tubes. One study showed no difference in failure rate (28% vs 35%) in patients receiving SBCTs (9 Fr) versus LBCTs (20–32 Fr).[22] In another study, the failure rate was 18% to 21% using SBCTs (5-Fr central venous catheters) or LBCTs (14–20 Fr).[23] The failure rate was 24% in patients who received a 7-Fr chest tube in another study.[24] Finally, 2 additional large retrospective studies showed failure rates of 12.5% to 15% with 8-Fr chest tubes[25] and 7% with 12-Fr chest tubes.[26] These studies were limited by their retrospective nature and incorporation of secondary spontaneous pneumothoraces. Regardless, the treating physician should be aware of the potential risk of failure with chest tube placement of any size.

Secondary spontaneous pneumothorax

Secondary spontaneous pneumothorax is caused by underlying lung abnormalities, including conditions such as bullous emphysema, cystic fibrosis, and *Pneumocystis pneumonia*. According to the BTS guidelines,[20] a secondary spontaneous pneumothorax larger than 2 cm or in symptomatic patients should undergo an SBCT placement. A smaller pneumothorax can be aspirated with a 16- or 18-gauge needle, although this cohort of patients should be admitted to the hospital and observed carefully while receiving supplemental oxygen.

In a retrospective review of 168 patients with secondary spontaneous pneumothorax, Chen and colleagues[27] reported the use of small-bore (10–16 Fr) pigtail catheters inserted using the trocar system. Patients on mechanical ventilation were excluded. Most patients (70%; n = 118) were successfully treated. Those that did not respond (30%; n = 50) underwent further management with either LBCT placement or video-assisted thoracoscopic surgery (VATS). The success rate was higher for patients with chronic obstructive pulmonary disease (COPD; 75%) and malignancy-associated pneumothorax (81%). The authors recommended treatment with LBCTs for infection-related secondary pneumothoraces related to Pneumocystis pneumonia and tuberculosis, and so forth, because less success was seen with smaller tubes (50%).

The BTS guidelines recommend consultation with a thoracic surgeon when an air leak persists for 48 hours after placement of a chest tube in patients with secondary pneumothorax.[20] In these patients, a persistent air leak may require VATS for underlying lung disease (eg, bullectomy), pleurodesis, or treatment with a Heimlich valve for a longer period before surgical intervention can be considered.

Traumatic pneumothorax

Although the data are scant, an increasing trend is occurring towards using SBCTs in the setting of a traumatic pneumothorax. One retrospective study compared the effectiveness of SBCTs and LBCTs in stable trauma patients.[28] Pneumothorax was the indication for 45% of the SBCTs and 69% of the LBCTs. Radiologists used image guidance (CT scan or ultrasound) to place small tubes (10–14 Fr; n = 131) using the Seldinger technique. Attending-supervised surgical residents placed large tubes without trocars (32–36 Fr; n = 71). Subsequent procedures were required in 14% of patients with SBCTs compared with 20% with LBCTs (*P* = not statistically significant). Complications included hemothorax (6% vs 4%) and empyema (3% vs 1%).

In another retrospective study of trauma patients over a 2-year period, 75 14-Fr pigtail catheters were placed for pneumothorax compared with 146 traditional chest tubes.[29] The tubes were inserted by surgery or emergency medicine physicians. The analysis noted a nonsignificant trend toward a higher tube failure rate in the pigtail catheter group compared with the chest tube group (11% vs 4%; *P* = .06). At this institution, small pigtail catheters were safe, able to be performed at the bedside, and became favored over traditional chest tube placement in the trauma setting for patients with pneumothorax. Additional prospective studies on chest tube size and character (pigtail vs straight) are required to make more definitive recommendations for patients with traumatic pneumothorax.

Pneumothorax in patients receiving mechanical ventilation

The type of chest tube required in patients on mechanical ventilation may depend on the cause of the pneumothorax. Traditionally, large-bore catheters have been favored because of the concern for an inability to evacuate large air leaks in patients receiving positive pressure ventilation. However, Lin and colleagues[30] reported their retrospective data on the management of 70 cases of pneumothorax in patients on mechanical ventilation. The authors reviewed placement of 12- to 16-Fr pigtail catheters inserted with ultrasound guidance via the Seldinger technique. The overall success rate was 68.6%; however, a significant difference in the success rate was seen among patients with iatrogenic- versus barotrauma-related pneumothorax. Management of iatrogenic pneumothoraces with pigtail catheters had 87.5% success rate compared with only 43.3% success in managing barotrauma-related pneumothoraces (P<.001).

Iatrogenic pneumothorax

Iatrogenic pneumothorax is seen with CT-guided transthoracic needle biopsies, bronchoscopy, thoracentesis, central venous line placement, and other procedures.[17,19] It can be treated with simple needle aspiration. However, SBCTs are very effective for managing these patients. A study by Galbois and colleagues[25] showed a low failure rate for small (8 Fr) chest tubes, with a second chest tube required in 11% and VATS in 2% of 130 patients with iatrogenic pneumothorax. Another study showed a failure rate of 2% in 48 patients with iatrogenic pneumothorax, which was similar whether SBCTs (5 Fr, Seldinger technique) or LBCTs (14–20 Fr, trocar technique) were used.[23] One study examined the management of pneumothorax related to image-guided transthoracic needle biopsy,[31] in which SBCTs (8.5 Fr) were used to treat 191 patients. Of these, 93% had immediate reexpansion of the lung and were treated as outpatients with a Heimlich valve, and only 9% needed additional interventions, such as a larger-sized tube.

Pleural Effusions

Malignant pleural effusions

Chest tubes are primarily used in malignant pleural effusion for symptom relief and chemical pleurodesis. Traditionally, LBCTs were used to instill a sclerosing agent to prevent blockage of the tube.[32] However, substantial evidence has shown that small-bore catheters can be used effectively for chemical pleurodesis.[17] The BTS guidelines recommend placement of an SBCT (10–14 Fr) for drainage and pleurodesis of malignant pleural effusion.[33] Indwelling pleural catheters are indicated for trapped lung in which pleurodesis is likely to be unsuccessful.[34] Various agents have been instilled via SBCTs when attempting chemical pleurodesis. In a prospective study by Patz and colleagues,[35] SBCTs (14 Fr) were inserted with image guidance using the Seldinger technique in 106 patients with malignant pleural effusions. Doxycycline was compared with bleomycin for achievement of pleurodesis, with similar success rates (43% for doxycycline and 40% for bleomycin). The same group showed a higher success rate (72%) using talc pleurodesis instilled through SBCTs.[36] In a separate

retrospective study examining chemical pleurodesis, 58 patients with SBCTs were compared with 44 patients with LBCTs.[37] Talc, doxycycline, bleomycin, and interferon alpha were used as sclerosing agents. The recurrence rate of the pleural effusion was similar (53% for SBCTs vs 51% for LBCTs) at 4 months, indicating no difference regardless of the size of chest tube chosen. A prospective study randomized 20 patients to receive LBCTs (32 Fr) and 23 to receive SBCTs for malignant effusions. Using iodopovidone as the sclerosing agent, the response rate was 90% for LBCTs and 87% for SBCTs at 3 months.[38]

A prospective, multicenter trial, the Second Therapeutic Intervention in Malignant Effusion trial (TIME2) recently compared patients undergoing talc pleurodesis using SBCTs (12 Fr) and those who received indwelling tunneled pleural catheters for management of their malignant effusions. Although the primary end point was dyspnea, an 89% success rate of pleurodesis was seen in the 54 patients who had talc slurry instilled via their SBCTs.[39] Similar outcomes were reported from another study.[40] These studies suggest that pleurodesis may be accomplished using SBCTs, while showing the efficacy of talc.

Parapneumonic effusion and empyema

The BTS guidelines recommend placement of a chest tube for empyema, complicated parapneumonic effusion with a pleural fluid pH less than 7.2, or multiloculated pleural effusions concerning for infection.[41] Despite the conventional practice of using LBCTs to drain thick purulent pleural fluid, the newest BTS recommendations support SBCTs (10–14 Fr) for empyema management when chest tubes are used. Ultrasound guidance for placement and routine flushing of the tubes are recommended.

The prospective, multicenter Multicenter Intrapleural Streptokinase Trial (MIST1) assessed the efficacy of intrapleural streptokinase in 405 patients with empyema or complicated parapneumonic effusion.[42] The primary outcome was the combined frequency of death and surgery, and secondary outcomes included length of hospital stay and change in chest radiograph and lung function at 3 months. No difference was seen in the percentage of patients who died or required surgery, regardless of the chest tube size placed for empyema (36%–44% with tubes <10 Fr and >20 Fr). Most of the small chest tubes were placed using the Seldinger technique and large ones were placed via blunt dissection. The secondary outcomes were also similar; however, patients who received larger tubes had significantly higher pain scores.

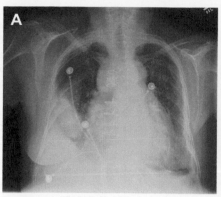
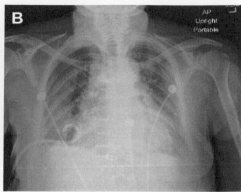

Fig. 6. Chest radiograph showing (*A*) loculated right pleural effusion. (*B*) The effusion resolved after placing a small pigtail chest tube.

In a recent prospective, multicenter, double-blind, randomized controlled MIST2 trial assessing the effectiveness of intrapleural tissue plasminogen activator (tPA) and DNase, most patients received SBCTs (<15 Fr).[43] A significant improvement in the pleural drainage, decreased surgical referral, and shorter hospital stay were seen in the group of patients that received tPA plus DNase as opposed to the groups not receiving combined treatment, showing the efficacy of dual therapy and supporting the use of small chest tubes for the initial management of empyema. Another study showed a 79% success rate using SBCTs (8–14 Fr) for drainage of empyema.[11] However, some studies have reported a higher failure rate with SBCTs.[26,44] Sometimes, image-guided small-bore catheters have been used when large bore tubes fail, especially for the drainage of loculated effusions (**Fig. 6**).[6,45]

Hemothorax

Hemothorax is the presence of blood in the pleural space, and is characterized by a pleural fluid hematocrit of at least 50% of the peripheral blood hematocrit. A chest tube is typically placed to quantify the rate of bleeding and to evacuate the pleural space. It may help to decrease the bleeding through apposition of parietal and visceral pleura.[17] Traditionally, LBCTs have been placed to facilitate drainage and prevent clots and thick fluid from inhibiting complete evacuation. However, SBCTs are increasingly placed successfully for patients with chest trauma, including those with hemothorax.[28,29]

Postoperative use of chest tubes

Since the description of their postoperative use by Lilienthal in 1922,[46] chest tubes are commonly placed during cardiothoracic surgical procedures to evacuate pleural effusions and pneumothorax (**Fig. 7**). Traditionally, LBCTs were used to prevent

clogging, because the tube blockage can lead to tension pneumothorax, inaccurate assessment of ongoing blood loss in the pleural space, and sepsis. However, small Blake drains (Ethicon Inc, Somerville, NJ, USA) are now being used because they are less painful and more flexible. The Blake drains are silicone tubes with a solid core center and 4 channels or flutes along the side. They exert constant suction over the entire length of the fluted portion of the drain, leading to efficient drainage of the fluid. They are connected to a pleural drainage unit with suction or water seal.

In a survey of 108 cardiothoracic surgeons and 108 nurses,[47] almost all surgeons observed chest tube clogging associated with adverse patient outcomes. Most surgeons (86%) reported that concern for clogging is why they use LBCTs. Approximately 70% of the surgeons would routinely place more than one large chest tube when clogging was anticipated. Only 33% used small-bore Blake drains routinely.

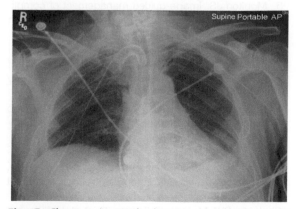

Fig. 7. Chest radiograph showing a straight LBCT placed during a surgical procedure (right lung transplant in a patient with a tracheostomy tube).

In a different study, 150 patients undergoing coronary artery bypass surgery were randomized to 24-Fr Blake drains or 32-Fr plastic or 32-Fr silastic chest tubes.[48] No tube was found to be superior, although all of these chest tubes were large-bore.

SUMMARY

Several types and sizes of chest tubes are available. Although chest tubes range in size (6–40 Fr) and shape (straight tubes vs pigtail catheters), small-bore tubes (<14 Fr) are effective for most pleural processes. Various types of pneumothorax and malignant and infected complicated pleural effusions have been successfully managed with SBCTs. Benefits of the smaller size include patient comfort and ease of placement. Most tubes can be placed using ultrasound guidance and the Seldinger technique. Although LBCTs may be necessary for barotrauma-associated pneumothoraces in mechanically ventilated patients and in the postoperative setting, abundant literature supports a paradigm shift towards the more routine use of SBCTs for managing pleural disease.

REFERENCES

1. Christopoulou-Aletra H, Papavramidou N. "Empyemas" of the thoracic cavity in the Hippocratic Corpus. Ann Thorac Surg 2008;85:1132–4.
2. Hewett FC. Thoracentesis: the plan of continuous aspiration. Br Med J 1876;1:317.
3. Havelock T, Teoh R, Laws D, et al. Pleural procedures and thoracic ultrasound: British thoracic Society pleural disease guideline 2010. Thorax 2010;65(Suppl 2):ii61–76.
4. Harris A, O'Driscoll BR, Turkington PM. Survey of major complications of intercostal chest drain insertion in the UK. Postgrad Med J 2010;86:68–72.
5. Moulton JS. Image-guided management of complicated pleural fluid collections. Radiol Clin North Am 2000;38:345–74.
6. vanSonnenberg E, Nakamoto SK, Mueller PR, et al. CT- and ultrasound-guided catheter drainage of empyemas after chest-tube failure. Radiology 1984;151:349–53.
7. Silverman SG, Mueller PR, Saini S, et al. Thoracic empyema: management with image-guided catheter drainage. Radiology 1988;169:5–9.
8. Grogan DR, Irwin RS, Channick R, et al. Complications associated with thoracentesis. A prospective, randomized study comparing three different methods. Arch Intern Med 1990;150:873–7.
9. Jones PW, Moyers JP, Rogers JT, et al. Ultrasound-guided thoracentesis: is it a safer method? Chest 2003;123:418–23.
10. Mayo PH, Goltz HR, Tafreshi M, et al. Safety of ultrasound-guided thoracentesis in patients receiving mechanical ventilation. Chest 2004;125:1059–62.
11. Shankar S, Gulati M, Kang M, et al. Image-guided percutaneous drainage of thoracic empyema: can sonography predict the outcome? Eur Radiol 2000;10:495–9.
12. Diacon AH, Brutsche MH, Soler M. Accuracy of pleural puncture sites: a prospective comparison of clinical examination with ultrasound. Chest 2003;123:436–41.
13. Fraser RS. Lung perforation complicating tube thoracostomy: pathologic description of three cases. Hum Pathol 1988;19:518–23.
14. Meisel S, Ram Z, Priel I, et al. Another complication of thoracostomy–perforation of the right atrium. Chest 1990;98:772–3.
15. Takanami I. Pulmonary artery perforation by a tube thoracostomy. Interact Cardiovasc Thorac Surg 2005;4:473–4.
16. Collop NA, Kim S, Sahn SA. Analysis of tube thoracostomy performed by pulmonologists at a teaching hospital. Chest 1997;112:709–13.
17. Light RW. Pleural controversy: optimal chest tube size for drainage. Respirology 2011;16:244–8.
18. Baumann MH, Patel PB, Roney CW, et al. Comparison of function of commercially available pleural drainage units and catheters. Chest 2003;123:1878–86.
19. Yarmus L, Feller-Kopman D. Pneumothorax in the critically ill patient. Chest 2012;141:1098–105.
20. MacDuff A, Arnold A, Harvey J. Management of spontaneous pneumothorax: British thoracic Society pleural disease guideline 2010. Thorax 2010;65(Suppl 2):ii18–31.
21. Baumann MH, Strange C, Heffner JE, et al. Management of spontaneous pneumothorax: an American College of Chest Physicians Delphi consensus statement. Chest 2001;119:590–602.
22. Vedam H, Barnes DJ. Comparison of large- and small-bore intercostal catheters in the management of spontaneous pneumothorax. Intern Med J 2003;33:495–9.
23. Contou D, Razazi K, Katsahian S, et al. Small-bore catheter versus chest tube drainage for pneumothorax. Am J Emerg Med 2012;30:1407–13.
24. Cho S, Lee EB. Management of primary and secondary pneumothorax using a small-bore thoracic catheter. Interact Cardiovasc Thorac Surg 2010;11:146–9.
25. Galbois A, Zorzi L, Meurisse S, et al. Outcome of spontaneous and iatrogenic pneumothoraces managed with small-bore chest tubes. Acta Anaesthesiol Scand 2012;56:507–12.
26. Cafarotti S, Dall'Armi V, Cusumano G, et al. Small-bore wire-guided chest drains: safety, tolerability, and effectiveness in pneumothorax, malignant

effusions, and pleural empyema. J Thorac Cardiovasc Surg 2011;141:683–7.

27. Chen CH, Liao WC, Liu YH, et al. Secondary spontaneous pneumothorax: which associated conditions benefit from pigtail catheter treatment? Am J Emerg Med 2012;30:45–50.

28. Rivera L, O'Reilly EB, Sise MJ, et al. Small catheter tube thoracostomy: effective in managing chest trauma in stable patients. J Trauma 2009; 66:393–9.

29. Kulvatunyou N, Vijayasekaran A, Hansen A, et al. Two-year experience of using pigtail catheters to treat traumatic pneumothorax: a changing trend. J Trauma 2011;71:1104–7 [discussion: 1107].

30. Lin YC, Tu CY, Liang SJ, et al. Pigtail catheter for the management of pneumothorax in mechanically ventilated patients. Am J Emerg Med 2010;28: 466–71.

31. Gupta S, Hicks ME, Wallace MJ, et al. Outpatient management of postbiopsy pneumothorax with small-caliber chest tubes: factors affecting the need for prolonged drainage and additional interventions. Cardiovasc Intervent Radiol 2008;31: 342–8.

32. Ruckdeschel JC, Moores D, Lee JY, et al. Intrapleural therapy for malignant pleural effusions. A randomized comparison of bleomycin and tetracycline. Chest 1991;100:1528–35.

33. Roberts ME, Neville E, Berrisford RG, et al. Management of a malignant pleural effusion: British thoracic Society pleural disease guideline 2010. Thorax 2010;65(Suppl 2):ii32–40.

34. Pien GW, Gant MJ, Washam CL, et al. Use of an implantable pleural catheter for trapped lung syndrome in patients with malignant pleural effusion. Chest 2001;119:1641–6.

35. Patz EF Jr, McAdams HP, Erasmus JJ, et al. Sclerotherapy for malignant pleural effusions: a prospective randomized trial of bleomycin vs .doxycycline with small-bore catheter drainage. Chest 1998;113: 1305–11.

36. Marom EM, Patz EF Jr, Erasmus JJ, et al. Malignant pleural effusions: treatment with small-bore-catheter thoracostomy and talc pleurodesis. Radiology 1999; 210:277–81.

37. Parulekar W, Di Primio G, Matzinger F, et al. Use of small-bore vs large-bore chest tubes for treatment of malignant pleural effusions. Chest 2001;120:19–25.

38. Caglayan B, Torun E, Turan D, et al. Efficacy of iodopovidone pleurodesis and comparison of small-bore catheter versus large-bore chest tube. Ann Surg Oncol 2008;15:2594–9.

39. Davies HE, Mishra EK, Kahan BC, et al. Effect of an indwelling pleural catheter vs chest tube and talc pleurodesis for relieving dyspnea in patients with malignant pleural effusion: the TIME2 Randomized Controlled Trial Indwelling Pleural Catheters vs Talc Pleurodesis. JAMA 2012;307:2383–9.

40. Fysh ET, Waterer GW, Kendall P, et al. Indwelling pleural catheters reduce inpatient days over pleurodesis for malignant pleural effusion. Chest 2012; 142:394–400.

41. Davies HE, Davies RJ, Davies CW. Management of pleural infection in adults: British thoracic Society pleural disease guideline 2010. Thorax 2010; 65(Suppl 2):ii41–53.

42. Rahman NM, Maskell NA, Davies CW, et al. The relationship between chest tube size and clinical outcome in pleural infection. Chest 2010;137:536–43.

43. Rahman NM, Maskell NA, West A, et al. Intrapleural use of tissue plasminogen activator and DNase in pleural infection. N Engl J Med 2011;365:518–26.

44. Horsley A, Jones L, White J, et al. Efficacy and complications of small-bore, wire-guided chest drains. Chest 2006;130:1857–63.

45. Westcott JL. Percutaneous catheter drainage of pleural effusion and empyema. AJR Am J Roentgenol 1985;144:1189–93.

46. Lilienthal H. Resection of the lung for suppurative infections with a report based on 31 operative cases in which resection was done or intended. Ann Surg 1922;75:257–320.

47. Shalli S, Saeed D, Fukamachi K, et al. Chest tube selection in cardiac and thoracic surgery: a survey of chest tube-related complications and their management. J Card Surg 2009;24:503–9.

48. Bjessmo S, Hylander S, Vedin J, et al. Comparison of three different chest drainages after coronary artery bypass surgery–a randomised trial in 150 patients. Eur J Cardiothorac Surg 2007;31:372–5.

Tunneled Pleural Catheters
An Update for 2013

Renelle Myers, MD, FRCPC[a], Gaetane Michaud, MD, FRCPC[b],*

KEYWORDS

- Pleural effusions • Tunneled pleural catheter • Lung cancer

KEY POINTS

- Tunneled pleural catheters (TPCs) are a safe, effective, and well-tolerated option for palliation in patients with malignant pleural effusion (MPEs) on an outpatient basis.
- TPCs are incorporated into international guidelines for the management of MPEs and appear to be the most cost-effective option according to current data.

Pleural effusions are commonly encountered in clinical practice, although the exact prevalence is unknown and is likely dependent on the population studied. When small or slowly accumulating, they may go unrecognized unless the patient undergoes chest imaging for some other clinical reason. Pleural effusions have been broadly grouped categorically into transudative and exudative effusions according to the criteria of Light and colleagues.[1] In brief, this classification is based on the integrity of the filtration barrier that is considered normal in transudative effusions and impaired in the case of exudates. As such, transudative effusions are usually of low protein content, whereas exudates contain a relatively high amount of protein. Most malignant and paramalignant effusions are exudative in nature, and the primary indication for the use of tunneled catheters is malignancy.

SYMPTOMS AND MANAGEMENT OPTIONS

In health, there exists a fine balance between the secretion and resorption of pleural fluid; however, in malignancy this homeostasis can become disrupted. As there is a large reserve in the ability to clear pleural fluid under normal conditions, there is usually both an increase in fluid production and an inability to maintain adequate removal

when effusions develop. Accumulation of fluid in the pleural space can lead to a myriad of symptoms including shortness of breath, cough, chest discomfort, and fatigue. It should be noted that many patients have several reasons for dyspnea, as well as for other pulmonary symptoms, during the course of their disease, and other causes of symptoms must be considered and addressed before definitive management of the pleural effusion. When effusion is the primary cause, symptoms are often relieved by removal of fluid from the pleural space, even in the context of a nonexpanding lung. In the particular case of "trapped lung," it is thought that the removal of fluid inhibits the stimulation of receptors in the hemithorax, in turn resulting in improvement in symptoms.

The impact on quality of life related to pleural effusions may be significant. Eighty-seven percent of new patients with lung cancer present with dyspnea, and 60% of patients with cancer grade their dyspnea as moderate to severe.[2,3] Dyspnea is the most common symptom associated with malignant pleural effusions (MPEs), and the majority of patients with MPEs are symptomatic. Once a patient is diagnosed with an MPE the life expectancy is typically 3 to 6 months, varying with the type of cancer. The general rule of thumb for MPE is recurrence.[4] Effusions related to breast

Disclosures: Dr Gaetane Michaud has no financial disclosures to make.
[a] RS 321 810 Sherbrooke Avenue, Winnipeg, Manitoba R3A 1R8, Canada; [b] 15 York Street, LCI 100, New Haven, CT 06510, USA
* Corresponding author.
E-mail address: Gaetane.michaud@yale.edu

chestmed.theclinics.com

cancer, small-cell lung cancer, hematologic malignancies, and other solid-organ tumor primaries will often respond to systemic therapies; therefore, definitive intervention beyond this approach may not be necessary. In this setting it is appropriate to proceed with simple drainage for symptomatic relief, pending response to the patient's systemic therapy. If, however, the pleural collection is refractory to systemic therapy, definitive management may be considered.

Talc pleurodesis and tunneled pleural catheters (TPCs) are the 2 most viable options for definitively dealing with MPEs. The decision to proceed with a TPC rather than pleurodesis depends on the patient's preference, whether the lung fully expands (necessary for pleurodesis), the patient's support systems, and other considerations. Definitive therapy should be considered once the patient becomes symptomatic to prevent trapped lung and loculation. Unfortunately, after drainage 30% of symptomatic patients with MPE do not achieve reexpansion of the lung adequate enough to allow an attempt at pleurodesis.[5] Of interest, small asymptomatic MPEs do not generally progress to the point of requiring intervention. In a 1-year study of 34 consecutive patients with known MPE from a large regional cancer center, 14 were asymptomatic.[6] These 14 patients were followed for their life span (median survival 128 days). Follow-up chest imaging was available in 13 of the 14 patients up to a median time of 98 days from first clinic visit. None of the follow-up images revealed an increase in the size of the effusions. No patient over the course of the study required pleural intervention for the index effusion. Of the patients studied, only 1 needed any subsequent intervention in the contralateral pleural space.

PATIENT SELECTION

A major advantage of the TPC as an option for treatment of MPE is the liberal patient selection. Performance status and operative risk have little impact on patient selection. Given that this patient population is at risk for multiple conditions leading to dyspnea (ie, lymphangitic carcinomatosis, anemia, radiation fibrosis, pulmonary embolus, pericardial disease, emphysema), often a therapeutic thoracentesis is performed before TPC insertion. Thoracentesis allows the provider to determine response to drainage, confirm whether the lung is able to reexpand, and assess how rapidly the effusion reaccumulates, if ever. If the lung is unable to reexpand sufficiently, few therapeutic options exists other than TPC. Decortication is infrequently performed for malignant lung entrapment, and an inability of the lung to adhere to the chest wall precludes successful pleurodesis. Conversely, there is no need for a TPC if the fluid does not reaccumulate following a large-volume thoracentesis or if symptoms are not improved by the procedure.

Patients with very short life expectancies (days to weeks) or those who are debilitated may be better served with other treatment options such as intermittent thoracentesis or nontunneled small-bore chest tubes. In these patients, the cost of intermittent drainage supplies and protection from pleural infection from a tunneled catheter may not confer any significant benefit. On the other hand, a TPC attached to a leg bag for continuous drainage is an inexpensive and well-tolerated method to achieve pleural drainage during the end stage of life. Other contraindications to TPC placement include coagulopathy, extensive malignant skin involvement (eg, inflammatory breast cancer), infection over the site of insertion, and multiloculated or septated effusions that would not drain even with a pleural catheter in place.

THE TUNNELED PLEURAL CATHETER SYSTEM

The TPC system is composed of a silicone catheter allowing ambulatory pleural drainage, on an intermittent basis, into plastic vacuum bottles. The catheter is composed of silicone with fenestrations at its distal margin (ie, the portion within the thoracic cavity) and a one-way valve on the proximal, external end for drainage purposes. A polyester cuff midway along the catheter acts as barrier to infection and promotes granulation tissue to secure the catheter in place. A special adapter is required to open the one-way valve at the proximal end of the catheter before drainage. This adapter is located on individual drainage lines and also on vacuum bottles specifically designed for this purpose. When the TPC is not being drained, a cap is placed over the one-way valve as an extra measure to ensure the valve remains clean and secure.

CATHETER PLACEMENT

Cather placement does not require inpatient admission and may be performed anywhere there is patient monitoring and a sterile environment; this may be in the intensive care unit, ambulatory procedure center, or operating room. Although topical anesthesia is standard, the type and dosages of other medications (such as intravenous analgesics or sedatives) varies.

There is no single ideal insertion site for all patients. Determinants of tube position include patient anatomy, location of the effusion by transthoracic ultrasonography, and patient comfort. Catheters should avoid breast tissue, excessive skin folds, undergarments, skin infection, and cutaneous tumor. It is preferable to avoid prior radiation fields, as the skin and soft tissues may be less amenable to tunneling of the catheter. Furthermore, lateral catheters may disrupt sleep for those who lie on their side. If the effusion is not loculated, positioning of the catheter just above the hemidiaphragm is optimal for drainage.

During placement, patients may be positioned semirecumbent with their ipsilateral arm over their head, or alternatively in the seated position with their arms crossed over a tray table, similar to during a thoracentesis. Patients may also be positioned in the lateral decubitus position with the affected side up. The best position depends on the clinical situation, operator preference, and patient factors already described.

In addition to physical examination, radiographic imaging may identify the most appropriate entry site. Ultrasonography can be particularly helpful in the setting of more complex fluid collections, metastatic involvement of the pleura, or the presence of adhesions. To avoid complications such as bleeding, it is best to avoid having the catheter traverse a metastatic deposit or breech an adhesion. In addition, ultrasonography allows the operator to confirm that he or she is indeed intrapleural and not in a subdiaphragmatic fluid collection.

The entry site is marked with a pen or by other indelible means. After preprocedural planning, the skin is cleansed with chlorhexidine over an extended surface that allows for a sterile margin around the catheter entry and exit sites, as well as along the entirety of the tunnel. Broad sterile drapes are applied, and additional drapes beyond those provided in the preprepared catheter kits are often necessary to ensure sterility throughout the procedure (**Box 1**). The operator dons personal protective wear including a hat, mask with face shield, sterile gown, and gloves. Lidocaine is used to inoculate the skin and soft tissues to the level of the parietal pleura and along the length of the tunnel site. Quantities as high as 40 mL of 1% lidocaine have been used routinely without complication. Of note, an entry site in the middle of the rib space as opposed to just above the rib is often selected to avoid kinking of the catheter on the rib. Bending of the catheter on the rib can lead to difficulties with drainage.

The track having been identified during the initial anesthesia, a guide needle with overlying sheath is then advanced while aspirating. Once a flash of pleural fluid is seen, the sheath is advanced into the pleural space and the needle removed (**Fig. 1**). A guide wire is passed through the sheath

---

> **Box 1**
> **List of supplies recommended for TPC insertion in addition to the supplied kit**
>
> *Required Supplies in Addition to TPC Insertion Kit:*
> - Antiseptic (chlorhexidine, povidone-iodine)
> - Personal protective equipment
> - Sterile drapes
> - Vacuum bottles or wall suction
> - Ultrasound

---

and into the pleural space, then the sheath is removed (**Fig. 2**). Two 1-cm incisions are made at the entry and exit sites, respectively (**Fig. 3**). The incision size should allow the catheter to fit tightly beneath the skin, minimizing the risk of dislocation of the catheter. The catheter is tunneled from the exit site toward the pleural entry site (ie, the site of the guide wire) (**Fig. 4**). The polyester cuff sits just beneath the skin at the exit site to allow for its access at the time of catheter removal. Thereafter, the entry site is dilated, the dilator and guide wire removed, and a peel-away sheath left in place. The catheter is rapidly advanced through the sheath to minimize the flow of air into the pleural space. Once the entire catheter has been advanced through the sheath, a thumb is placed over the silicone tubing and the sheath peeled apart and removed (**Fig. 5**). The exit site is closed and the catheter secured in place with suture material.

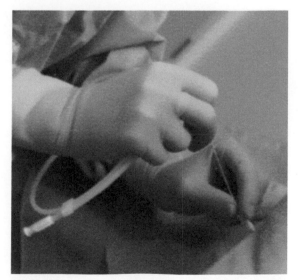

Fig. 1. A guide wire is advanced into the pleural space.

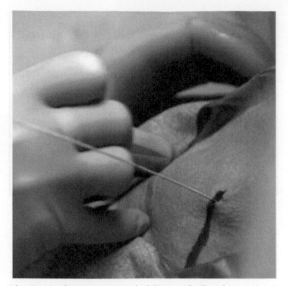

Fig. 2. Catheter is tunneled beneath the skin.

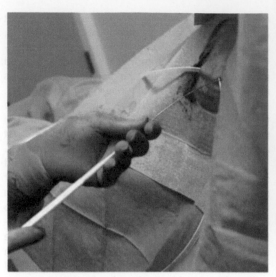

Fig. 4. A dilator is advanced over the guide wire into the pleural space.

Once the catheter is secured, the pleural space is drained. The drainage line is connected to the one-way valve at the end of the TPC and pleural drainage is initiated into a wall suction apparatus or vacuum bottle. Pleural fluid is removed as tolerated until a maximum volume is achieved or the patient develops symptoms such as cough, pain, or dyspnea. The drainage system is then disconnected and the plastic valve cap provided is clicked onto the valve. The incisions are sutured and a dressing applied. A foam drain sponge may be placed over both incisions with the catheter through the central opening and curled over the sponge. The sponge and catheter may then

be covered by 2 to 4 layers of gauze and a self-adhesive water-resistant dressing (Fig. 6). A chest radiograph is typically performed following catheter insertion to ensure adequate placement and lack of complications. Once the radiograph is reviewed by the physician, the patient may be discharged home.

ROUTINE CATHETER DRAINAGE

Supplies for drainage are ordered in bulk for ongoing drainage. Typically the packages include

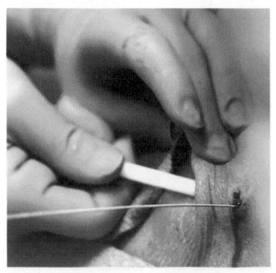

Fig. 3. Catheter is tunneled beneath the skin.

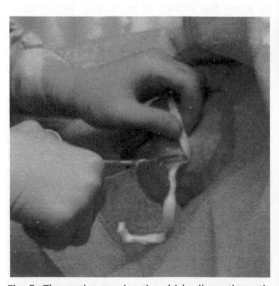

Fig. 5. The peel-away sheath, which allows the catheter to be introduced, is removed after catheter insertion.

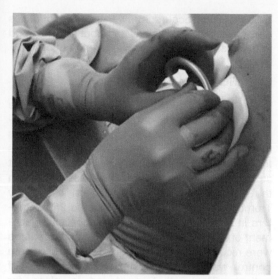

Fig. 6. The catheter is coiled upon itself to allow for dressing application.

gloves, sterile supplies, dressings, and drainage bottles (500 mL and 1 L). At present, the standard of care is to drain the catheter intermittently, either on alternate days or 3 times weekly. On rare occasions when patients are producing large volumes of fluid on a daily basis, the frequency of drainage is increased to daily, or a leg bag is connected to the catheter to decrease costs and the need for frequent drainage procedures. In a current multi-center study, patients are being randomized to daily versus intermittent drainage to test the hypothesis that daily drainage improves symptom management and results in more rapid eradication of the pleural space. As suggested earlier, the amount of fluid that can be drained varies significantly between patients. Removal of volumes as high as 1 L has been shown to be safe, and does not require volume repletion with colloids or crystalloids. In select cases where patients have bilateral catheters, more attention to volume shifts may be necessary. Drainage is discontinued when the flow stops, indicating an evacuated space, or when the patient becomes symptomatic. Some patients complain of chest tightness and others of refractory cough when they reach their symptomatic limit, although symptoms depend on the individual. Persistence of drainage beyond the onset of symptoms may result in protracted discomfort on the part of the patient, and is not advised.

ONGOING CARE OF THE PATIENT WITH A TPC

Patients with indwelling tunneled catheters benefit from continuity of care and accessibility to a team experienced in not only insertion but also the long-term management of these devices. This goal often is achieved in the context of multidisciplinary teams with one or more chest physicians, oncology and palliative care providers, skilled nursing personnel, mid-level practitioners, and family members or friends. The patient and others specially trained in the management of tunneled catheters perform the chronic management of the catheter. Ideally patients and their families receive training on the method of catheter drainage, application of dressings, sterile technique, and indications for reaching health care providers if problems arise. When the patient is not in a facility or home nursing is not arranged, initial education may include videos, reading materials, and observation of drainage by members of the health care team.

A routine follow-up visit is generally scheduled for all patients 2 weeks after insertion. At this time, a radiograph is performed and symptoms, concerns and complications are addressed. The incisions are inspected and sutures are removed if not done by the home care team. Patients are then seen on an as-needed basis if problems or new symptoms arise, or if catheter removal is indicated.

DISCONTINUATION OF THE TPC

The effusions stops accumulating, or pleurodesis occurs, in approximately 50% of patients who have a TPC placed for malignancy. The rate of spontaneous pleurodesis is higher in patients whose lungs fully reexpand following catheter insertion, suggesting the importance of maintaining pleural apposition and minimizing residual fluid in the pleural space. In these cases, the catheter can be removed because it is no longer serving its purpose, and to avoid infection from having a foreign body in place.

The authors' criterion for catheter removal is drainage of less than 50 mL on 3 consecutive attempts in the absence of increasing symptoms or an accumulating effusion on radiography. Catheter removal does not require hospitalization or intravenous medications. Typically the skin surrounding the exit site is cleansed, and approximately 5 mL of 1% lidocaine is infiltrated around the tissue cuff with a 25-gauge needle. The catheter is then withdrawn by applying a steady and firm traction on the catheter with a circular motion. Occasionally small forceps may be required to free the cuff from the subcutaneous tissues. Steri-strips and a dry dressing are applied to the exit site. On occasion, a significant amount of pleural fluid drains from the site following removal of the TPC, likely from loculated fluid pockets near the insertion site. The authors have managed this by applying an ileostomy system over the incision to contain the fluid, which can usually be removed within 48 hours as drainage stops.

COMPLICATIONS

TPC placement and maintenance is safe and free of complications in the vast majority of patients. Complications include infections, clogging of the catheter, or other rare events. Empyema can occur in 1% to 5% of patients, usually late in the course of treatment.[7,8] Empyema has been successfully treated using a combination of intravenous antibiotics and continuous pleural drainage through the TPC. In certain circumstances, additional small-bore chest tubes or thrombolytics for loculated infections may be necessary. The TPC can be removed once the infection has resolved, as the pleural space usually achieves symphysis secondary to inflammation from the infection. Cellulitis has been reported in up to 7% of patients,[8] but has been lower in the authors' experience (1.4%). Cellulitis is usually an early event and responds to oral antibiotics without the need for catheter removal.

Patients often notice fibrin deposits partially occluding the tube. These deposits will often clear spontaneously during drainage, and rarely occlude the TPC itself. However, they may block the drainage line. In rare cases, the tube may need to be flushed with sterile saline and then aspirated to dislodge the fibrin. Before flushing the tube, it may be prudent to attempt a second drainage with a new bottle, as failure to drain may be attributable to loss of suction in the first bottle.

Significant bleeding necessitating catheter removal is rare, although fluid drained is often bloody in appearance. The hematocrit of the fluid can be measured, but is rarely found to be elevated and should not be considered the sole cause for anemia in most patients. In addition, a recent article by Fysh and colleagues[9] described fracture of the catheters on removal. Fortunately, none of the patients described had any significant negative effects related to the portion of the catheter remaining in situ.

There exist patients who have failed attempts at catheter insertion, develop loculated fluid collections, or develop recurrence after removal of the catheter. If symptomatic loculations occur while the TPC is still in place, administration of thrombolytics may facilitate drainage. Ultrasound-guided placement of a new catheter into large loculations may ameliorate dyspnea and therefore may be considered. Finally, extrapleural extension of the tumor through the insertion site can be seen.

This extension occurs in fewer than 3% of cases and is rarely clinically significant, but may respond to local radiation treatment if symptomatic.

EVIDENCE FOR USE OF TPC

TPC placement allows for the safe and effective palliation of MPE in an outpatient setting. Management of symptoms as an outpatient allows patients to maintain control over their lives and minimizes time spent in the hospital. The first and largest study demonstrating the effectiveness of TPCs in the palliation of MPE was published in 2006 by Tremblay and Michaud,[8] who placed 250 catheters in 223 patients. Following successful placement of the TPC, no further ipsilateral procedures were required in 90% of the cases and symptom control was partial or complete in 88.8% of patients. The catheters stayed in place for a median duration of 56 days. Spontaneous pleurodesis occurred at a rate of 42.9% in all patients, and when the population was limited to those whose lungs fully reexpanded following catheter insertion, the rate was in the range of 60%.

A systematic review published in 2010 by Van Meter and colleagues[7] included 19 reports comprising a total of 1370 patients. Symptom improvement was noted in 95.6% of patients and spontaneous pleurodesis in 45.6%, allowing for catheter removal in 47.1% of those patients. Recurrence of the effusion after catheter removal ranged from 5.1% to 7.7%. The reports included in the review were consecutive case series with the exception of one randomized trial. The review concluded that TPCs are safe and that prospective randomized studies comparing the TPC with pleurodesis are needed before recommending TPC as first-line therapy.

One study comparing TPC with talc pleurodesis included 106 patients randomized to receive an outpatient TPC versus hospital admission for placement of a 12F percutaneous chest tube and talc pleurodesis.[10] The primary outcome was dyspnea at 42 days. The study concluded that both methods are highly effective at relieving dyspnea, and no significant difference was identified in the frequency of chest pain or quality of life. A reduction in hospital stay and improved dyspnea were noted as secondary outcomes 6 months postprocedure in the TPC group. There was also a 16% absolute reduction in the proportion of patients requiring further pleural interventions in the TPC group. In light of the limited life span of patients with pleural effusions, TPCs show promise in requiring fewer hospital days, improving dyspnea, and decreasing the need for additional procedures.[11]

As described earlier, lung reexpansion must be considered when determining prospects for pleurodesis. In the case of patients with nonexpanding lungs, TPCs remain one of the sole options for palliation of dyspnea related to recurrent malignant effusions. A survey of patients with nonexpanding lungs demonstrated that nearly 50% were either very or moderately satisfied with their symptomatic relief following insertion of a TPC.[11] Of note, it is suggested to stop drainage at the onset of chest discomfort to avoid pain associated with drainage of a nonexpanding lung, as pain can persist for several hours to days in this scenario.

Hybrid approaches using TPC insertion at the same time as thoracoscopic talc pleurodesis have been proposed.[12] In this study, a TPC was placed under direct thoracoscopic guidance immediately following talc poudrage. A 24F chest tube was inserted into the port site and maintained for 24 hours to ensure resolution of pneumothorax. The TPC was drained 3 times on the first postoperative day, twice daily on days 2 and 3, and then daily until less than 150 mL was drained. The intent of this approach was to reduce the number of days in the hospital after thoracoscopy, as well as to reduce the time that the patient maintains the TPC. This pilot study for rapid pleurodesis included 31 patients. The mean duration of hospital stay was 3.19 (standard deviation [SD] 3.04) days, and the TPC was removed at a mean of 16.65 (SD 30.8) days. Successful pleurodesis occurred in 92% of the patients at 6 months. The rapid pleurodesis approach allows for most patients to be discharged home in 48 hours and have the TPC removed in 2 weeks, thus giving them the benefits of a shorter admission than for conventional thoracoscopic pleurodesis and freedom from prolonged tunneled catheter drainage. Additional studies are required.

TPCS IN MESOTHELIOMA

Pleural effusions are common in malignant mesothelioma (MM), and methods to relieve the associated respiratory symptoms are important in this incurable disease. The most common procedure for palliation of symptomatic effusions in this setting has traditionally been talc pleurodesis. Recently, TPC insertion has also been described. A single-center retrospective review included 26 patients treated with 31 TPCs.[13] Complete or partial symptom control was obtained in 93.5% of patients and spontaneous pleurodesis occurred in 38.7%. Seeding of the catheter tract was not reported as a complication, although it does remain a concern in MM. If this was to occur, it could be managed effectively with local radiation therapy to the site.

TPCS IN CHYLOTHORAX

Chylothorax in patients with cancer is difficult to manage, and primary treatment is focused on the underlying malignancy. Unfortunately, in patients with poor or no response chylothorax may become debilitating by causing significant dyspnea. There is a paucity of data regarding the use of TPCs in this setting. The largest review compared 19 patients with malignant chylothorax: 10 treated with a TPC and 9 by other palliative measures.[14] All patients with a TPC had symptom relief and 60% of the patients achieved pleurodesis. Ongoing drainage did cause a decrease in serum albumin, but was not significantly different to that in patients undergoing other palliative procedures.

TPCS AND BENIGN DISEASE

Although there are case reports and case series documenting the usage of TPC in the palliation of end-stage benign diseases such as heart failure and hepatic hydrothorax, there are insufficient data to be able to comment on their efficacy and long-term safety at present.

COST-EFFECTIVENESS OF TPC FOR MPE

Because of the ongoing expense of the drainage system and the need for home care, cost is considered a potential barrier to the placement of TPCs; this holds particularly true for patients unable to self-drain and who have no available friends or family to assist. In this scenario, the cost burden includes supplies but also visiting care providers. However, Olden and Holloway[15] showed that the overall cost-effectiveness of TPCs was equivalent to that of pleurodesis via a talc slurry. The cost and effectiveness of the modalities were reported as follows: talc $8170.80 and 0.281 quality-adjusted life years (QALYs); TPC $9011.60 and 0.276 QALYs. In patients with a limited life expectancy (ie, $\leq$6 weeks), TPC placement was found to be more cost-effective. The greatest limitations of this analysis are that the investigators used a simple model and considered talc pleurodesis via slurry as the only alternative to TPC. Many centers perform pleurodesis via thoracoscopy rather than slurry, and this was not analyzed. With respect to the simple nature of the model, it did not consider the ongoing costs of care and, in particular, the impact when the palliative attempts fail. The model assumed that patients did not receive modalities that accrued cost or affected quality of life beyond the initial modality. An abstract presented by the authors at the American Thoracic Society (ATS) international conference in 2011 compared the cost benefit of talc pleurodesis by video-assisted thoracoscopic surgery (VATS), medical thoracoscopy (MT), and talc slurry (TS) with that of TPCs.[16] TPCs were the most cost-effective at $1958/quality-adjusted life month (QALM) and dominated the other 3 options: $19,149 per QALM for VATS, $9844/QALM for MT, and $8737/QALM for TS. Sensitivity analyses failed to identify factors associated with significant changes in cost-effectiveness. This model did consider potential failures and was iterative in nature. A subsequent study by Puri and colleagues[17] also suggested that TPCs are the preferred treatment for patients with MPE and limited survival. As such, the available cost-benefit data would suggest that tunneled catheters do provide a cost-effective means to palliate symptomatic patients with malignant effusions, particularly so when life expectancy is short and protracted draining periods are unlikely.

SUMMARY

TPCs are a safe, effective, and well-tolerated option for palliation in patients with MPEs on an outpatient basis. TPCs are incorporated into international guidelines for the management of MPEs and appear to be the most cost-effective option according to current data.

REFERENCES

1. Light R, Macgregor I, Luchsiner PC, et al. Pleural effusions: the diagnostic separation of transudates and exudates. Ann Intern Med 1972;77:507–13.
2. Hollen PJ, Gralla RJ, Kris M, et al. Normative data and trends in quality of life from the Lung Cancer Symptom Scale (LCSS). Support Care Cancer 1999;7:140–8.
3. Viola R, Kiteley C, Lloyd N, et al. The management of dyspnea in cancer patient: a systematic review. Support Care Cancer 2008;16:329–37.
4. Robert ME, Neville E, Berrisford R, et al. Management of a malignant pleural effusion: British Thoracic Society pleural disease guideline 2010. Thorax 2010;65(Suppl 2):ii32–40.
5. Dresler CM, Olak J, Herndon JE, et al. Phase III intergroup study of talc poudrage vs talc slurry sclerosis for malignant pleural effusion. Chest 2005;127:909–15.
6. Tremblay A, Robbins S, Berthiaume L, et al. Natural history of asymptomatic pleural effusions in lung cancer patients. Journal of Bronchology 2007;14(2):98–100.
7. Van Meter ME, McKee KY, Kohlwes RJ. Efficacy and safety of tunneled pleural catheters in adults with malignant pleural effusions: a systematic review. J Gen Intern Med 2011;26:70–6.
8. Tremblay A, Michaud G. Single-center experience with 250 tunnelled pleural catheter insertions for malignant pleural effusion. Chest 2006;129:362–8.
9. Fysh ET, Wrightson JM, Lee YC. Fractured indwelling pleural catheters. Chest 2012;141(4):1090–4.
10. Davies H, Mishra E, Kahan BC, et al. Effect of an indwelling pleural catheter vs chest tube and talc pleurodesis for relieving dyspnea in patients with malignant pleural effusions. The TIME2 Randomized Controlled Trial. JAMA 2012;307(22):2383–9.
11. Efthymiou CA, Masudi T, Thorpe JA, et al. Malignant pleural effusion in the presence of trapped lung. Five-year experience of PleurX tunnelled catheters. Interact Cardiovasc Thorac Surg 2009;9:961–4.
12. Reddy C, Ernst A, Lamb C, et al. Rapid pleurodesis for malignant pleural effusions: a pilot study. Chest 2010;139:1419–23.
13. Tremblay A, Patel M, Michaud G. Use of tunneled pleural catheters in malignant mesothelioma. J Bronchol 2005;12:203–6.
14. Jimenez CA, Mhatre AD, Martinez CH, et al. Use of an indwelling pleural catheter for the management of recurrent chylothorax in patients with cancer. Chest 2007;132:1584–90.
15. Olden A, Holloway R. Treatment of malignant pleural effusion: PleuRx® catheter or talc pleurodesis? A cost-effectiveness analysis. J Palliat Med 2010;13(1):59–65.
16. Michaud G, Ryder H, Ankrom A, et al. Cost effectiveness analysis of strategies for managing malignant pleural effusions. Am J Respir Crit Care Med 2011;183:A3082.
17. Puri V, Pyrdeck TL, Crabtree TD, et al. Treatment of malignant pleural effusion: a cost-effective analysis. Ann Thorac Surg 2012;94(2):374–9.

Pleuroscopy in 2013

Pyng Lee, MD, FCCP[a,*], Henri G. Colt, MD, FCCP[b]

KEYWORDS

- Thoracoscopy • Pleural effusion • Video-assisted thoracoscopic surgery (VATS) • Pleuroscopy

KEY POINTS

- Pleuroscopy is effective in the evaluation of pleural and pulmonary diseases when routine fluid analysis and cytology fail.
- In many institutions where facilities for thoracoscopy are available, it replaces second-attempt thoracentesis and closed needle biopsy for patients with exudative effusions of unclear etiology.
- Pleuroscopy also offers the nonsurgeon the ability to intervene therapeutically.
- Although pleuroscopy is generally safe, it is still an invasive procedure, and to minimize complications, training in techniques and instrumentation is required.
- The flex-rigid pleuroscope is a significant invention in the era of minimally invasive pleural procedures and is likely to replace traditional biopsy methods in the future.
- The future will continue to define the "when and how" to use flex-rigid and rigid instruments when evaluating a variety of pleural diseases.

Thoracoscopy, medical thoracoscopy, pleuroscopy, and video-assisted thoracic surgery (VATS) are terms that are used interchangeably to describe a minimally invasive procedure that provides the physician a window to the pleural space, differing only in the approach to anesthesia. In this article, the primary focus is medical thoracoscopy (pleuroscopy).

VATS refers to a thoracoscopic procedure performed in the operating room using single-lung ventilation with double-lumen endotracheal intubation, 3 entry ports, and rigid instruments. Stapled lung biopsy, resection of pulmonary nodules, lobectomy, pneumonectomy, esphagectomy, and pericardial windows are performed with VATS, in addition to guided parietal pleural biopsy, drainage of pleural effusion or empyema, and pleurodesis (**Table 1**).[1,2] Medical thoracoscopy, or pleuroscopy, refers to thoracoscopy typically conducted by a nonsurgeon pulmonologist in an endoscopy suite with the patient under local

anesthesia and conscious sedation. Pleuroscopy is an endoscopic procedure that examines the pleural cavity, facilitates drainage of pleural fluid, and guides parietal pleural biopsy, talc pleurodesis, and chest tube placement without endotracheal intubation and general anesthesia.[3] Some practitioners in Europe perform pleuroscopic sympathectomy for essential hyperhidrosis, and lung biopsy for diffuse lung disease.[4]

Thoracoscopy was documented in a report dated 1866 when Richard Cruise examined the pleural space of an 11-year-old girl with empyema.[5] Thoracoscopy did not gain widespread use until Hans Christian Jacobaeus published his technique, also known as the Jacobaeus operation, in 1910.[6] He created a pneumothorax by severing adhesions using galvanocautery that collapsed the underlying lung, thereby allowing safe entry, as well as an unobstructed examination of the pleural space. He strongly advocated thoracoscopic-guided biopsies for pleural effusions of indeterminate

Disclosures: The authors have no financial disclosures.
[a] Division of Respiratory & Critical Care Medicine, Department of Medicine, Yong Loo Lin Medical School, National University Hospital, National University of Singapore, 1E Kent Ridge Road, NUHS Tower Block Level 10, Singapore 119228; [b] Division of Pulmonary and Critical Care Medicine, Irvine Medical Center, University of California, CA, USA
* Corresponding author.
E-mail address: mdclp@nus.edu.sg

chestmed.theclinics.com

Table 1
VATS versus medical thoracoscopy (pleuroscopy)

Procedure	VATS	Medical Thoracoscopy (Pleuroscopy)
Where	OR	Endoscopy suite or OR
Who	Surgeons	Trained nonsurgeons
Anesthesia	General anesthesia Double lumen intubation Single lung ventilation	Local anesthesia Conscious sedation Spontaneous respiration
Indications	Parietal pleural biopsy, pleurodesis, decortication, stapled lung biopsy, lung nodule resection, lobectomy, pneumonectomy, pericardial window, esophagectomy lung	Parietal pleural biopsy, pleurodesis, chest tube placement under direct visualization

Abbreviations: OR, operating room; VATS, video-assisted thoracic surgery.

etiology, and applied thoracoscopy as both a diagnostic and therapeutic tool.[7]

EQUIPMENT
Rigid Instruments

Historically, rigid endoscopic instruments, such as stainless steel trocars and telescopes, have been pivotal in the technique.[4,8,9] Trocars come in different sizes (5–13 mm diameter) and are made of disposable plastic or reusable stainless steel. These trocars have changed little over time, but operators have increasingly moved to disposable, plastic, ribbed trocars with either plastic or steel inner cannulas. Rigid telescopes have different angles of vision. Thoracoscopy performed by rigid endoscopic equipment requires a cold (xenon) light source, an endoscopic camera attached to the eyepiece of the telescope, and a video monitor and recorder (**Fig. 1**). The O-degree telescope is useful for direct viewing, whereas the oblique (30-degree or 50-degree) and periscope (90-degree) telescopes offer a panoramic view of the pleural cavity. Selection of the optimal trocar size and telescope depends on the operator's preferences and patient considerations. A large trocar that accommodates a larger telescope with better optics improves the quality of exploration; however, compression of the intercostal nerve during manipulation of the trocar can cause greater discomfort, especially if the procedure is performed under local anesthesia and conscious sedation. We prefer the 7-mm trocar, the direct viewing (0-degree) 4-mm or 7-mm telescope, and the 5-mm optical forceps that allow pleural biopsies without a second puncture site.

Sowemaller telescopes and instruments have also been used. Tassi and Marchetti[10] reported excellent views of the pleural space using a 3.3-mm telescope for a group of patients with small, loculated pleural effusions that were inaccessible to standard-sized instruments. Two 3.8-mm trocars were used: one for the 3.3-mm telescope and the other for 3-mm biopsy forceps. The reported diagnostic yield of 93.4% was comparable with that achieved using conventional 5-mm biopsy forceps.

Flex-rigid Pleuroscope

A single 1-cm skin incision that accommodates a disposable flexible trocar should suffice for the flex-rigid pleuroscope. The flex-rigid pleuroscope (model LTF 160 or 240, Olympus, Tokyo, Japan) is fashioned like the flexible bronchoscope. It consists of a handle and a shaft that measures 7 mm in outer diameter and 27 cm in length. The shaft is made up of a 22-cm proximal rigid portion and 5-cm flexible distal end. The flexible tip is movable by a lever on the handle, which allows 2-way angulation (160 degrees up and 130 degrees down). It has a 2.8-mm working

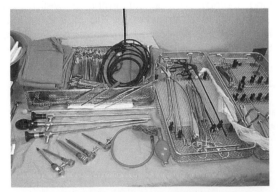

Fig. 1. Rigid trocars, telescopes, and accessories.

channel that accommodates biopsy forceps, needles, and other accessories, and is compatible with various electrosurgical and laser procedures (**Fig. 2**). The LTF 160 model also allows autoclaving.[11] A notable advantage of the flex-rigid pleuroscope over rigid instruments is its easy interface with existing processors (CV-160, CLV-U40) and light sources (CV-240, EVIS-100 or 140, EVIS EXERA-145 or 160). These are made by the same manufacturer for flexible bronchoscopy or gastrointestinal endoscopy and are therefore available in most endoscopy units at no additional cost.[3,12]

INDICATIONS AND CONTRAINDICATIONS FOR PLEUROSCOPY

Although the only absolute contraindication for medical thoracoscopy is the lack of a pleural space because of adhesions, this can be overcome by enlarging the skin incision or digitally dissecting the lung away from the chest wall. As thoracoscopy is performed under conscious sedation in a spontaneously breathing patient with partial or near-total lung collapse, these patients must not have respiratory insufficiency requiring mechanical ventilation, intolerable hypoxemia unrelated to the pleural effusion, an unstable cardiovascular status, bleeding diathesis, refractory cough, or allergy to the medications used.

PATIENT PREPARATION

A detailed history and physical examination are vital components of any preoperative evaluation. The chest radiograph (CXR), decubitus films, ultrasonography (US), and computed tomography (CT) scan aid in the selection of the appropriate entry site. Before pleuroscopy, approximately 200 to 300 mL of fluid is typically aspirated from the pleural cavity using a needle, angiocatheter, thoracentesis catheter, or Boutin pleural puncture needle. This is followed by induction of a pneumothorax by opening the needle to air until stable

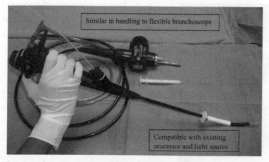

Fig. 2. Pleuroscope within flexible trocar and flexible biopsy forceps (LTF 160/240, Olympus).

equilibrium is achieved. Air causes the lung to collapse away from the chest wall, thereby creating a space for trocar insertion. Conversely, the operator may choose to do the procedure directly with the aid of US.[13]

ANESTHESIA

Benzodiazepines (midazolam) combined with opioids (demerol, fentanyl, morphine) provide adequate analgesia and sedation.[14] Meticulous care toward administration of local anesthesia to the 4 layers (epidermis, aponeurosis, intercostal muscles, and parietal pleura at the entry site) ensures patient comfort during manipulation of the thoracoscope.[15] There is a trend in recent years toward greater use of propofol to enhance patient comfort if talc poudrage is planned; however, this requires monitoring by anesthesiologists in many countries.[16] We have successfully performed thoracoscopic talc poudrage for pneumothoraces and malignant effusions using benzodiazepines and opioids and anesthetizing the pleura before talc poudrage with 250 mg of 1% lidocaine with a spray catheter.[17] Preoperative anesthesia is individualized to the patient's general condition and the advantages and disadvantages of various methods for pain control are carefully considered.

TECHNIQUE

The patient is first placed in the lateral decubitus position with the affected side up and the arm above the head. The patient's vital parameters, electrocardiogram, blood pressure, and oxygenation by means of pulse oximetry are monitored. A single-port access located between the fourth and seventh intercostal spaces of the chest wall and along the midaxillary line should suffice for diagnostic pleuroscopy, guided pleural biopsy, and talc poudrage. A second port might be necessary to facilitate adhesiolysis, drainage of complex loculated fluid collections, lung biopsy, or sampling of pathologic lesions located around the first entry site. Similarly, double-port access may be necessary to evaluate the pleural space completely when the rigid telescope is used, especially if the posterior and mediastinal aspects of the hemithorax are inaccessible because of partial collapse of lung, or when the lung parenchyma is adherent to the chest wall. With the flex-rigid pleuroscope, only a single port is required because its nimble tip allows easy maneuverability within a limited pleural space and around adhesions.[11,12,17,18] At the end of diagnostic thoracoscopy, a chest tube is inserted and air is aspirated. The tube can be removed as soon as the lung has reexpanded, and the patient may be discharged after a brief observation in a recovery area. If talc pleurodesis or lung biopsy is performed, the patient is hospitalized for a period of monitoring and chest tube drainage.

Thoracoscopic-Guided Biopsy of Parietal Pleura

Biopsy of the parietal pleura should be performed over a rib to avoid the neurovascular bundle. This can be achieved with the rigid optical or flexible forceps (**Fig. 3**). The forceps are first used to probe the rib and to feel the hard undersurface, followed by grasping of the overlying parietal pleura and removing of the pleura with a long tearing rather than a "grab-and-pull" motion. Specimens that are obtained with the rigid forceps are significantly larger than those with Abram or Cope needle. Biopsies with the flex-rigid pleuroscope are small, as they are limited by size of the flexible forceps, which in turn depend on the diameter of the working channel. The flexible forceps also lack mechanical strength in obtaining pleural specimens of sufficient depth, a major factor that affects yield when mesothelioma is suspected. This technical hitch can be overcome by taking multiple biopsies (range: 5–10) of the abnormal areas as well as several "bites" of the same area to obtain tissue of sufficient depth.

Electrosurgical Biopsy of Parietal Pleura

Electrocautery has been incorporated with the flexible forceps biopsy to enhance its yield. Full-thickness parietal pleural biopsies can be achieved using the insulated tip (IT) diathermic knife during flex-rigid pleuroscopy. In one study, the reported diagnostic yields were 85% with IT knife, compared with 60% with flexible forceps. The IT knife was notably useful when smooth,

thickened lesions were encountered, of which nearly half were malignant mesothelioma.[19]

Management of Hemorrhage

The principal danger in performing pleural biopsies is hemorrhage from the inadvertent biopsy of an intercostal vessel. Immediate external application of finger pressure at the site of bleeding in the intercostal space is the first intervention. During this time, another incision is made to provide additional access to the pleural cavity. The physician can use 2 separate entry sites to examine the bleeding area while cauterizing the tissues. Direct pressure can also be applied from the inside, using a gauze peanut mounted on a forceps. Reexpansion of the lung by connecting a chest tube to underwater seal aids in providing tamponade to the bleeding site. Very rarely, if bleeding does not abate with these measures, the thoracic surgeon might have to ligate the bleeding vessels with endoclips, enlarge the incision to facilitate repair, or even consider thoracotomy.

Thoracoscopic Talc Poudrage

Chemical pleurodesis plays an integral role in the management of malignant effusions, as most recur unless the primary tumor is chemosensitive. Similarly, one of the primary goals in secondary spontaneous pneumothorax management is recurrence prevention. Chemical pleurodesis can be performed via instillation of sclerosants through intercostal tubes or small-bore catheters, or via talc poudrage during thoracoscopy. A *Cochrane Database Systematic Review* of pleurodesis for malignant effusions, which includes 36 randomized controlled trials consisting of 1499 patients, supports talc as the sclerosant of choice and thoracoscopic talc poudrage as the preferred technique for all patients with good performance status (**Fig. 4**).[20] Thoracoscopic talc poudrage can be performed following fluid aspiration and

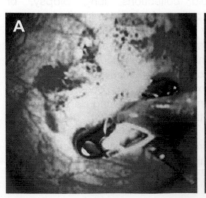 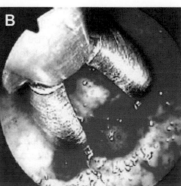

Fig. 3. Forceps biopsy of parietal pleura with (*A*) flexible forceps and (*B*) rigid optical forceps.

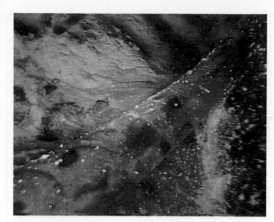

Fig. 4. Thoracoscopic talc poudrage.

pleural biopsy. Various delivery devices are available, such as a talc spray atomizer, a bulb syringe, or a spray catheter introduced through the working channel of the flex-rigid pleuroscope.

COMPLICATIONS

Mortality from conventional thoracoscopy using rigid instruments ranges between 0.09% and 0.24%,[21,22] which is comparable to that associated with bronchoscopic transbronchial lung biopsy. Complications caused by thoracoscopy are listed in **Box 1**.

Complications with the flex-rigid pleuroscope, on the other hand, are rare. In fact, it has been shown to be very safe when performed by trained pulmonologists.[11,18] We previously reported our safety and outcome results in 51 patients with indeterminate pleural effusions who underwent flex-rigid pleuroscopy. No morbidity or mortality was observed[18]; however, studies of complication rates typically involve procedures performed by

specialists and may not reflect circumstances with less experienced physicians. The need for adequate and satisfactory training cannot be overemphasized. **Table 2** describes the type of patient suitable for rigid or flex-rigid pleuroscopy.

CLINICAL APPLICATIONS FOR PLEUROSCOPY
Pleural Effusion of Unknown Etiology

The first step toward investigating pleural effusion is thoracentesis. More than half of exudative effusions are attributable to malignancy,[23] and although pleural fluid cytology is the simplest definitive method, its diagnostic yield depends on the extent of disease and nature of the primary malignancy.[24] Cytologic examination of the pleural fluid may be positive in 62% of patients with metastatic disease[24] and in fewer than 20% for mesothelioma.[25] Repeated large-volume thoracentesis increases the yield by 27% with a second aspiration, and a further 5% with a third.[26] The addition of closed pleural biopsy merely improves the yield by 10%, and is of little value for tumors confined to the diaphragmatic, visceral, or mediastinal pleura.[27]

In effusions in which the cause is unknown, additional radiography may be beneficial. Contrast-enhanced CT is better than standard CT for the evaluation of the pleura, and features such as nodularity, irregularity, and pleural thickness greater than 1 cm are highly suggestive of malignancy.[28,29] Imaging of the pleura can be performed at the patient's bedside using US, and US is increasingly used to guide pleural procedures, particularly in the selection of appropriate sites for thoracentesis, tube thoracostomy, and thoracoscopy.[13] Certain US features, such as pleural thickening of more than10 mm, pleural nodularity, and diaphragmatic thickening of more than 7 mm, are diagnostic of malignancy, with 73% sensitivity and 100% specificity.[30] An "echogenic swirling pattern," characterized by numerous free-floating echogenic particles swirling in the pleural cavity during respiratory movement or heartbeat, is another sign indicative of malignant pleural effusion.[31] Although these CT and US features may suggest pleural metastasis, histology is still the gold standard, and where pleuroscopy is not readily available, image-guided pleural biopsy is an alternative. In one study, CT-guided needle biopsy achieved an 87% yield, compared with 47% using the Abram needle, when parietal pleura measured more than 5 mm. US-guided biopsy of pleural lesions measuring more than 20 mm with a 14-gauge cutting needle demonstrated comparable yield to CT (85.5%), even for malignant mesothelioma, with a 4% rate of pneumothorax.[32]

Box 1
Complications of pleuroscopy

- Prolonged air leak
- Hemorrhage
- Subcutaneous emphysema
- Postoperative fever
- Empyema
- Wound infection
- Cardiac arrhythmias
- Hypotension
- Seeding of chest wall from mesothelioma

Table 2
Indications for rigid or semi-rigid pleuroscopy

Clinical Scenario	Type of Procedure
Diagnostic thoracoscopy for indeterminate, uncomplicated pleural effusion where suspicion of mesothelioma is not high	Flex-rigid pleuroscopy[a] or use of rigid telescopes under local anesthesia
Trapped lung with radiographically thickened pleura	Rigid optical biopsy forceps[a] or flex-rigid pleuroscopy with flexible forceps performing multiple bites over the same area to obtain specimens of sufficient depth or use of flexible forceps and IT knife
Mesothelioma is suspected	Rigid optical biopsy forceps[a] or flex-rigid pleuroscopy with IT knife
Pleuro-pulmonary adhesions	Fibrous: Rigid optical biopsy forceps[a] or flex-rigid pleuroscopy with electrocautery accessories Thin, fibrinous: flex-rigid pleuroscopy with flexible forceps
Empyema, split pleural sign, loculated pleural effusion	Rigid instruments (VATS)[a] or conversion to thoracotomy for decortication
Pneumothorax with bulla or blebs	Rigid instruments (VATS)[a] for staple bullectomy

Abbreviations: IT, insulated tip; VATS, video-assisted thoracic surgery.
  [a] Denotes procedure preferred.

Despite repeated thoracentesis and image-guided needle biopsy, 20% of pleural effusions remain undiagnosed.[33] The primary advantage of thoracoscopy is to enhance our diagnostic capabilities when other minimally invasive tests fail.[34] If a neoplasm is strongly suspected, the diagnostic sensitivity of thoracoscopic exploration and biopsy approaches 90% to 100%.[8–12,14,18] Certain endoscopic characteristics, such as nodules, polypoid masses, and "candle wax drops," are highly suggestive of malignancy (see **Fig. 4**); however, early-stage mesothelioma can resemble pleural inflammation (**Fig. 5**).[33,34] Additional image modalities may supplement pleuroscopic evaluation. Janssen and coworkers[35] added autofluorescence to white light thoracoscopy for the evaluation of 24 patients with exudative pleural effusions. The aims were to determine if the autofluorescence mode could differentiate early malignant lesions from nonspecific inflammation, aid in selecting appropriate sites for biopsy, and better delineate tumor margins for more precise staging. A color change from white/pink to red was demonstrated in all cases of malignant pleuritis (sensitivity: 100%). These lesions were more easily located and their margins more precisely delineated with autofluorescence thoracoscopy. In 2 cases of chronic pleuritis, a color change from white/pink to orange/red was also observed, giving a specificity of 75%. Although the investigators concluded that there was little value of autofluorescence thoracoscopy in clinical practice, as most patients with malignant pleural effusions had extensive pleural involvement that was easy to diagnose with white light thoracoscopy, the autofluorescence mode might be useful when early

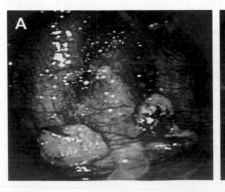
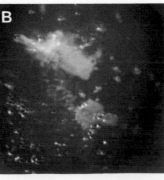

Fig. 5. Endoscopic findings of (*A*) polypoid masses and (*B*) candle wax nodules.

pleural malignancies are studied.[35] Similar conclusions were derived from a recent study that evaluated narrow band imaging (NBI) incorporated into the flex-rigid videopleuroscope (prototype Olympus XLTF 160). NBI technology uses unfiltered narrow bands in the blue (415 nm) and green (540 nm) light wavelengths that coincide with the peak absorption of oxyhemoglobin. By applying these wavelengths, NBI enhances the vascular architecture of tissues. In this study, all patients had malignant involvement of the pleura, of which 9 were mesothelioma. The investigators did not find a difference in the diagnostic accuracy between NBI and white light videopleuroscopy (**Fig. 6**).[36] We have had similar observations in 45 patients with pleural effusions of unclear etiology (Lee et al, 2012). In our cohort, 32 patients had pleural metastases, 12 had pulmonary tuberculosis, and 1 had chronic pleuritis, and all patients were followed for 12 months. Although NBI enhanced the pleural vasculature well, it was difficult to discriminate tumor neovascularization from inflammation based on vascular patterns. In patients with metastatic pleural malignancy, NBI demarcated tumor margins clearly, but there was no difference in the quality of biopsies obtained with white light versus NBI.

Baas and coworkers[37] investigated if prior administration of 5-aminolaevulinic acid (ALA) before VATS could lead to the improved detection and staging of thoracic malignancy. In this study, patients were given 5-ALA by mouth 3 to 4 hours before VATS. The pleural cavity was then examined using white light followed by fluorescence thoracoscopy (D Light Autofluorescence System, Karl Storz Germany). Tissue sampling of all abnormal areas was performed, and histologic diagnoses were compared against thoracoscopic findings. The fluorescence mode did not provide a superior diagnostic accuracy over white light, but led to upstaging in 4 of 15 patients with mesotheliomas owing to better visualization of visceral pleural

lesions that were otherwise undetectable by white light. Several postoperative complications were reported, but the investigators concluded that fluorescence thoracoscopy using 5-ALA was feasible with minimal side effects, and it could have potential applications in the diagnosis and staging of mesothelioma.

Lung Cancer

Cancer-related pleural effusions occur as a result of direct tumor invasion, tumor emboli to the visceral pleura with secondary seeding of the parietal pleura, hematogenous spread, or via lymphatic involvement. Elastin staining and careful examination for invasion beyond the elastic layer of the visceral pleura should be performed for lung cancer resections, as visceral pleural invasion is regarded as an important stage-defining feature in the absence of nodal involvement. Metastatic spread of lung cancer to the pleura adversely affects survival, and in the recent TNM staging of lung cancer, presence of pleural metastasis is defined as M1a (from T4), representing a corresponding change from stage IIIB to stage IV.[38] It is rare to find resectable lung cancer in the setting of an exudative pleural effusion, despite negative cytologic examination. Thus, pleuroscopy can establish operative eligibility by determining if the pleural effusion is paramalignant or due to metastases.[23] If pleural metastases are found, and therefore confirming inoperable disease, talc poudrage can be performed at the same setting. This has been shown to be more effective in preventing recurrence than intrapleural instillation of a sclerosant.[20]

Malignant Mesothelioma

The average survival of a patient diagnosed with malignant mesothelioma is 6 to 18 months, and death often occurs from respiratory failure.[39] Malignant mesothelioma is atop the differential

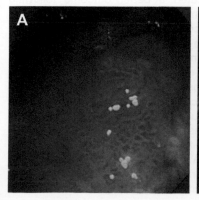
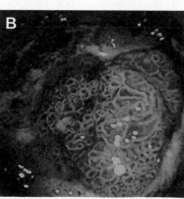

Fig. 6. (*A*) White light versus (*B*) narrow-band imaging of pleural metastasis due to breast cancer.

diagnosis in a patient with a history of asbestos exposure and characteristic radiographic findings of a pleural effusion without contralateral mediastinal shift. Diagnosis by pleural fluid cytology and closed needle biopsy is often difficult, which has prompted some physicians to advocate open biopsy by mini or lateral thoracotomy to obtain specimens of sufficient size and quantity for immunohistochemical stains and electron microscopy.[40] Pleural fluid mesothelin (>2 nmol/L) and megakaryocyte potentiating factor (MPF; >12.4 ng/mL), which originate from a common precursor protein, have shown 65% sensitivity and 95% specificity for pleural mesothelioma in a large study consisting of 507 patients.[41]

Pleuroscopy is favored over thoracotomy, as the pleural specimens obtained with 5-mm or 7-mm rigid forceps are comparable with open biopsies.[42] Pleuroscopy allows staging to be performed in a minimally invasive manner, and fluorescence detection using 5-ALA is a method to improve its staging accuracy.[37] Adequacy of the tissue obtained with the flexible forceps is a valid concern, and as such, we recommend the rigid 5-mm optical forceps or IT knife for biopsy in cases in which mesothelioma is suspected.[19,43] Mesothelioma is notorious for seeding biopsy and chest tube sites, thus pleuroscopy and chest tube incisions should be chosen to allow for excision if subsequent therapeutic resection is performed. Consideration should also be given to prophylactic irradiation.[44] Only 5% of patients are suitable for curative surgery.[45] As such, a palliative approach with aggressive palliation of dyspnea by removing pleural fluid or performing talc poudrage, providing a focus on improved pain control, and performing prophylactic irradiation of incision sites, have conferred good symptom control.[46]

Tuberculous Pleural Effusion

The diagnostic yield from closed needle biopsy in tuberculous (TB) pleural effusions is variable (28%–88%).[47] In a prospective study of 100 TB effusions in Germany, an immediate histologic diagnosis was established by pleuroscopy in 94%, compared with 38% by closed needle biopsy (**Fig. 7**). A positive yield from tissue cultures was also found to be higher with pleuroscopic-guided biopsies than with closed needle biopsy tissue and pleural fluid combined.[48] In another study of TB-endemic countries, thoracoscopic-guided pleural biopsies achieved superior yield over closed needle biopsies with the Abram needle (98% vs 80%). Pleuroscopy has a role where large quantities of pleural tissue are required for

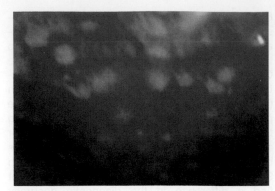

Fig. 7. Sago nodules in a tuberculous effusion.

culture in suspected drug-resistant cases, and for adhesiolysis to promote drainage of fluid loculations.[49]

Empyema and Complicated Parapneumonic Effusions

For pulmonologists intent on performing pleuroscopy for management of empyema, the procedure should be conducted early in the course of disease.[50,51] Lysis of thin fibrinopurulent adhesions and guided chest tube placement during pleuroscopy may facilitate fluid drainage and hasten clinical resolution. When the "split pleural sign" is observed on CT, however, it suggests the presence of a thick pleural peel, trapped lung, or complicated multiloculated pleural space. This finding should prompt surgical referral for decortication.[52]

Pneumothorax

In spontaneous pneumothorax (SP), thoracoscopy can reveal blebs and bullae. These can be coagulated and SP recurrence prevented by pleural abrasion or talc pleurodesis. Detection of blebs and bullae is higher with VATS or thoracotomy than pleuroscopy[53]; however, investigators have not demonstrated a better outcome following specific treatment of bullae associated with primary or secondary SP.[54,55] This is particularly relevant to the group of patients with secondary SP from advanced lung disease. These patients are at higher risk of general anesthesia, VATS, and thoracotomy, but require interventions to prevent SP recurrence. In these patients, pleuroscopic talc poudrage performed under local anesthesia and conscious sedation has been shown to be an effective therapeutic option.[17,56] In recurrent primary SP, VATS with staple bullectomy and parietal pleural abrasion, pleurectomy, or talc poudrage is preferred.[57]

Pleuroscopic Lung Biopsy

Forceps lung biopsies have been used by pulmonologists in the evaluation of patients with diffuse lung disease, especially if the diagnoses are not achieved by bronchoscopic bronchoalveolar lavage and transbronchial lung biopsy.[58] Its application has decreased because of improvement in imaging techniques, such as high-resolution CT, and the increasing use of VATS for wedge lung biopsy.[59]

Pleuroscopic Sympathectomy

Thoracoscopic sympathectomy for essential hyperhidrosis is typically performed by surgeons using the 3-entry port technique, general anesthesia, and single-lung and double-lumen ventilation, whereas the thoracic sympathetic chain is interrupted at level T3. There has been a trend toward a simplified, bilateral approach using clipping or diathermy cauterization, single-lumen intubation, and smaller-diameter trocars. This procedure can be safely performed by trained interventional pulmonologists.[60]

SUMMARY

Pleuroscopy is effective in the evaluation of pleural and pulmonary diseases when routine fluid analysis and cytology fail. In many institutions where facilities for thoracoscopy are available, it replaces second-attempt thoracentesis and closed needle biopsy for patients with exudative effusions of unclear etiology. Pleuroscopy also offers the non-surgeon the ability to intervene therapeutically: to break down loculations in early empyemas and complicated parapneumonic effusions, and to perform pleurodesis for recurrent malignant effusions and pneumothoraces. Although pleuroscopy is generally safe, it is still an invasive procedure, and to minimize complications, training in techniques and instrumentation is required.[61,62] The flex-rigid pleuroscope is a significant invention in the era of minimally invasive pleural procedures and is likely to replace traditional biopsy methods in the future.[63] The future will continue to define the "when and how" to use flex-rigid and rigid instruments when evaluating a variety of pleural diseases.

REFERENCES

1. McKenna RJ Jr. Thoracoscopic evaluation and treatment of pulmonary disease. Surg Clin North Am 2002;80:1543–53.
2. Yim AP, Lee TW, Izzat MB, et al. Place of video-thoracoscopy in thoracic surgical practice. World J Surg 2001;25:157–61.
3. Lee P, Mathur PN, Colt HG. Advances in thoracoscopy: 100 years since Jacobaeus. Respiration 2010;79:177–86.
4. Tassi GF, Davies RJ, Noppen M. Advanced techniques in medical thoracoscopy. Eur Respir J 2006;28:1051–9.
5. Moisiuc FV, Colt HG. Thoracoscopy: origins revisited. Respiration 2007;74:344–55.
6. Jacobaeus HC. Uber die Moglichkeit, die Zystoskopie bei Untersuchungen seroser Hohlungenanzuwenden. Munch Med Wochenschr 1910;40:2090–2.
7. Jacobaeus HC. The practical importance of thoracoscopy in surgery of the chest. Surg Gynecol Obstet 1922;34:289–96.
8. Rodriguez-Panadero F, Janssen JP, Astoul P. Thoracoscopy: general overview and place in the diagnosis and management of pleural effusion. Eur Respir J 2006;28:409–21.
9. Colt HG. Thoracoscopy: window to the pleural space. Chest 1999;107:1409–15.
10. Tassi G, Marchetti G. Minithoracoscopy: a less invasive approach to thoracoscopy-minimally invasive techniques. Chest 2003;124:1975–7.
11. Munavvar M, Khan MA, Edwards J, et al. The autoclavable semi-rigid thoracoscope: the way forward in pleural disease? Eur Respir J 2007;29:571–4.
12. Lee P, Colt HG. State of the art: pleuroscopy. J Thorac Oncol 2007;2:663–70.
13. Hersh CP, Feller-Kopman D, Wahidi M, et al. Ultrasound guidance for medical thoracoscopy: a novel approach. Respiration 2003;70:299–301.
14. Mathur P, Astoul P, Boutin C. Medical thoracoscopy. Clin Chest Med 1995;16:479–86.
15. Migliore M, Giuliano R, Aziz T, et al. Four-step local anesthesia and sedation for thoracoscopic diagnosis and management of pleural diseases. Chest 2002;121:2032–5.
16. Danby CA, Adebonojo SA, Moritz DM. Video-assisted talc pleurodesis for malignant pleural effusions utilizing local anesthesia and IV sedation. Chest 1998;113:739–42.
17. Lee P, Colt HG. A spray catheter technique for pleural anesthesia: a novel method for pain control before talc poudrage. Anesth Analg 2007;104:198–200.
18. Lee P, Hsu A, Lo C, et al. Prospective evaluation of flex-rigid pleuroscopy for indeterminate pleural effusion: accuracy, safety and outcome. Respirology 2007;12:881–6.
19. Sasada S, Kawahara K, Kusunoki Y, et al. A new electrocautery pleural biopsy technique using an insulated-tip diathermic knife during semirigid pleuroscopy. Surg Endosc 2009;23:1901–7.

20. Shaw P, Agarwal R. Pleurodesis for malignant pleural effusions. Cochrane Database Syst Rev 2004;(1):CD002916.

21. Viskum K, Enk B. Complications of thoracoscopy. Poumon Coeur 1981;37:25–8.

22. Boutin C, Viallat JR, Cargnino P. La thoracoscopie en 1980. Revue generale. Poumon Coeur 1981;37:11–9.

23. American Thoracic Society. Management of malignant pleural effusions. Am J Respir Crit Care Med 2000;162:1987–2001.

24. Hsu C. Cytologic detection of malignancy in pleural effusion: a review of 5,255 samples from 3,811 patients. Diagn Cytopathol 1987;3:8–12.

25. Renshaw AA, Dean BR, Antman KH, et al. The role of cytologic evaluation of pleural fluid in the diagnosis of malignant mesothelioma. Chest 1997;111:106–9.

26. Starr RL, Sherman ME. The value of multiple preparations in the diagnosis of malignant pleural effusions: a cost-benefit analysis. Acta Cytol 1991;35:533–7.

27. Canto A, Ferrer G, Ramagosa V, et al. Lung cancer and pleural effusion: clinical significance and study of pleural metastatic locations. Chest 1985;87:649–51.

28. Leung AN, Mueller NL, Miller RR. CT in differential diagnosis of diffuse pleural disease. AJR Am J Roentgenol 1990;154:487–92.

29. Traill ZC, Davies RJ, Gleeson FV. Thoracic computed tomography in patients with suspected malignant pleural effusions. Clin Radiol 2001;56:193–6.

30. Qureshi NR, Rahman NM, Gleeson FV. Thoracic ultrasound in the diagnosis of malignant pleural effusion. Thorax 2009;64:139–43.

31. Chian CF, Su WL, Soh LH, et al. Echogenic swirling pattern as a predictor of malignant pleural effusions in patients with malignancies. Chest 2004;126:129–34.

32. Diacon AH, Schuurmans MM, Theron J, et al. Safety and yield of ultrasound-assisted transthoracic biopsy performed by pulmonologists. Respiration 2004;71:519–22.

33. Boutin C, Cargnino P, Viallat JR. Thoracoscopy in the early diagnosis of malignant pleural effusions. Endoscopy 1980;12:155–60.

34. Weissberg D, Kaufman M, Zurkowski Z. Pleuroscopy in patients with pleural effusion and pleural masses. Ann Thorac Surg 1980;29:205–8.

35. Chrysanthidis MG, Janssen JP. Autofluorescence videothoracoscopy in exudative pleural effusions: preliminary results. Eur Respir J 2005;26:989–92.

36. Schonfeld N, Schwarz C, Kollmeier J, et al. Narrow band imaging (NBI) during medical thoracoscopy: first impressions. J Occup Med Toxicol 2009;4:24–8.

37. Baas P, Triesscheijn M, Burgers S, et al. Fluorescence detection of pleural malignancies using 5-aminolaevulinic acid. Chest 2006;129:718–24.

38. Rami-Porta R, Crowley JJ, Goldstraw P. The revised TNM staging system for lung cancer. Ann Thorac Cardiovasc Surg 2009;15:4–9.

39. Ceresoli GL, Locati LD, Ferreri AJ, et al. Therapeutic outcome according to histologic subtype in 121 patients with malignant pleural mesothelioma. Lung Cancer 2001;34:279–87.

40. Legha SS, Muggia FM. Pleural mesothelioma: clinical features and therapeutic implications. Ann Intern Med 1977;87:613–21.

41. Herbert A, Gallagher PJ. Pleural biopsy in the diagnosis of malignant mesothelioma. Thorax 1982;37:816.

42. Hollevoet K, Nackaerts K, Thimpont J, et al. Diagnostic performance of soluble mesothelin and megakaryocyte potentiating factor in mesothelioma. Am J Respir Crit Care Med 2010;181:620–5.

43. Boutin C, Rey F. Thoracoscopy in pleural malignant mesothelioma: a prospective study of 188 consecutive patients. Part 1. Diagnosis. Cancer 1993;72:389–93.

44. Boutin C, Rey F, Viallat JR. Prevention of malignant seeding after invasive diagnostic procedures in patients with pleural mesothelioma: a randomized trial of local therapy. Chest 1995;108:754–8.

45. Sugarbaker DJ, Garcia JP, Richards WG, et al. Extrapleural pneumonectomy in the multimodality therapy of malignant pleural mesothelioma. Results in 120 consecutive patients. Ann Surg 1996;224:288–94.

46. Parker C, Neville E. Management of malignant mesothelioma. Thorax 2003;58:809–13.

47. Mathur PN, Loddenkemper R. Medical thoracoscopy: role in pleural and lung diseases. In: Beamis JF Jr, Mathur PN, editors. Interventional pulmonology. New York: McGraw-Hill Inc; 1999. p. 169–84.

48. Loddenkemper R, Mai J, Scheffeler N, et al. Prospective individual comparison of blind needle biopsy and of thoracoscopy in the diagnosis and differential diagnosis of tuberculous pleurisy. Scand J Respir Dis 1978;102:196–8.

49. Diacon AH, Van de Wal BW, Wyser C, et al. Diagnostic tools in tuberculosis pleurisy: a direct comparative study. Eur Respir J 2003;22:589–91.

50. Cameron RJ. Management of complicated parapneumonic effusions and thoracic empyema. Intern Med J 2002;32:408–14.

51. Colice GL, Curtis A, Deslauriers J, et al. Medical and surgical treatment of parapneumonic effusions: an evidence-based guideline. Chest 2000;18:1158–71.

52. Heffner JE, Klein JS, Hampson C. Interventional management of pleural infections. Chest 2009;136:1148–59.

53. Lee P, Colt HG. Thoracoscopy: an update on therapeutic applications. J Respir Dis 2003;24:530–6.

54. Schramel FM, Postmus PE, Vanderschueren RG. Current aspects of spontaneous pneumothorax. Eur Respir J 1997;10:1372–9.

55. Tschopp JM, Boutin C, Astoul P, et al. Talcage by medical thoracoscopy for primary spontaneous pneumothorax is more cost-effective than drainage: a randomized study. Eur Respir J 2002;20:1003–9.

56. Lee P, Yap WS, Pek WY, et al. An audit of medical thoracoscopy and talc poudrage for pneumothorax prevention in advanced chronic obstructive pulmonary disease. Chest 2004;125:1315–20.

57. Baumann MH, Strange C, Heffner JE, et al. Management of spontaneous pneumothorax: an American College of Chest Physicians Delphi Consensus Statement. Chest 2001;119:590–602.

58. Vansteenkiste J, Verbeken E, Thomeer M, et al. Medical thoracoscopic lung biopsy in interstitial lung disease: a prospective study of biopsy quality. Eur Respir J 1999;14:585–90.

59. Loddenkemper R, Mathur PN, Noppen M, et al, editors. Medical thoracoscopy/pleuroscopy. Manual and atlas. Stuttgart (Germany), New York: Thieme; 2011.

60. Noppen M, Herregodts P, D'Haese J, et al. A simplified T2-T3 sympathicolysis technique for the treatment of essential hyperhidrosis: short-term results in 100 patients. J Laparoendosc Surg 1996;6:151–9.

61. Konge L, Lehnert P, Hansen HJ, et al. Reliable and valid assessment of performance in thoracoscopy. Surg Endosc 2012;26:1624–8.

62. Colt HG, Davoudi M, Quadrelli S, et al. Use of competency based metrics to determine effectiveness of a post-graduate thoracoscopy course. Respiration 2010;80:553–9.

63. Lee P, Colt HG. Steps to flex-rigid pleuroscopy. In: Lee P, Colt HG, editors. Flex-rigid pleuroscopy: step by step. Singapore: CMP Medica Asia; 2005. p. 77–111.

Thoracoscopy: A Real-Life Perspective

Frank C. Detterbeck, MD

KEYWORDS

- Video-assisted thoracic surgery • Thoracoscopy • Pleuroscopy

KEY POINTS

- It is clear that some pleural conditions are more straightforward and lend themselves more easily to being managed by practitioners with a variety of backgrounds, if they have the interest and acquire the necessary skills.
- Management of more complex pleural infections requires more experience and judgment.
- How care is delivered depends on many different factors in a particular institution, and there is no simple answer that fits all situations. The value of a dedicated interest in organizing the care process and proactively working to make it better is crucial.
- Exceptional care requires a team that works together seamlessly.

INTRODUCTION

Thoracoscopy, commonly known as video-assisted thoracic surgery (VATS), refers to the use of a camera and optics to visualize the inside of the chest and carry out diagnostic and therapeutic thoracic procedures. There is some variation in what this means beside the use of a video camera. Some have referred to procedures performed only with video camera and visualization on a monitor as a complete VATS. Some have used the term VATS-assisted for procedures in which the camera is used as an adjunct, with at least part of the surgical procedure being performed with direct visualization of intrathoracic structures through a small (limited thoracotomy) incision.[1] However, there is consensus that the term thoracoscopy should be applied to procedures performed through a small incision, without any rib spreading, with essentially all of the procedure being performed with visualization via a monitor.[2,3]

For all practical purposes, thoracoscopy began to be implemented in the late 1980s, although its roots can be traced back many decades earlier. In the early 1990s, thoracoscopy had evolved to be used for major procedures such as lobectomy.[4] However, although it had become standard to perform minor procedures via thoracoscopy, for a variety of reasons, major thoracoscopic resections were performed infrequently until about a decade later. This situation was partly because of resistance to change and the learning curve, especially among older practitioners, and partly because there was a lack of significant outcomes data for resection of lung cancer via VATS until around 2000.

However, since then, there have been many studies, enough to summarize in systematic reviews and meta-analyses.[5–9] These studies have all shown that compared with open thoracotomy, VATS has a lower rate of morbidity and mortality and shorter hospital lengths of stay. Furthermore, for lung cancer, long-term outcomes have been equivalent.[5–8,10] This benefit comes at a minor cost of about 20 minutes longer operative times for anatomic lung resection (eg, lobectomy) by VATS. Most of these data come from nonrandomized comparative studies, but are corroborated by randomized studies, case-matched analyses, and large database outcomes studies.[11–15]

VATS lobectomy is becoming the standard of care for early-stage lung cancer, according to the third edition of the *American College of Chest Physicians Lung Cancer Guidelines*. Although only

Disclosures: None.
Department of Thoracic Surgery, Yale University School of Medicine, 330 Cedar Street, BB205, New Haven, CT 06520-8062, USA
E-mail address: frank.detterbeck@yale.edu

Clin Chest Med 34 (2013) 93–98
http://dx.doi.org/10.1016/j.ccm.2012.12.002

about 25% of lobectomies in the United States are performed via VATS, in the centers that perform VATS, most major lung resections are performed this way.[10,16] The VATS approach has been extended to procedures such as segmentectomy, pneumonectomy, sleeve resections, lobectomy with en-bloc chest wall resection, and even extrapleural pneumonectomy for mesothelioma.[6,17–20]

The focus of this issue of *Clinics in Chest Medicine* is pleural disease, and therefore the rest of this article is restricted to thoracoscopy for pleural procedures, both diagnostic and therapeutic. For a well-referenced article on medical thoracoscopy (pleuroscopy) in the management of pleural disease, please see that by Pyng and Colt elsewhere in this issue. The present article examines whether there is a real difference between pleuroscopy and thoracoscopy or VATS and how thinking should be structured regarding management of pleural disease in the modern context of available approaches and interventions.

IS THERE A DIFFERENCE BETWEEN PLEUROSCOPY AND THORACOSCOPY?

From a semantic perspective, pleuroscopy refers to visualization of the pleural space and pleural surfaces, whereas thoracoscopy is more generic, referring to visualization of essentially anything in the chest. However, because this article is restricted to thoracoscopy for pleural procedures, it is unclear whether in this context, there is a difference semantically.

Probably the most common distinction between the 2 refers to the background of the person performing the procedure. Thoracoscopy is used primarily when the intervention is performed by someone who has had formal surgical training, whereas (medical) pleuroscopy is used when performed by someone with primary internal medicine training. However, given the need for additional training among those with a major focus on interventional thoracic procedures, and the evolution of a more disease-based and organ-based multispecialty team approach to care, the future appropriateness of traditional divisions in medicine and training is highly questionable. If the distinction is a matter of who performs the procedure, a more transparent and straightforward description is provided by terms such as thoracoscopy performed by a thoracic surgeon or thoracoscopy performed by an interventional pulmonologist.

However, the background of the person performing the procedure is probably important in determining the extent and complexity of pleural interventions with which they are comfortable or that they should be apprehensive about getting involved with. This discussion should go beyond medical versus surgical training roots and include many other aspects, such as whether the individual has a focus on thoracic versus general or cardiac surgery, has a focus on pleural procedures, and has experience with the increasing number of technologies available for pleural interventions.

Sometimes thoracoscopy and pleuroscopy are differentiated by whether the procedure is performed under general anesthesia or local anesthesia and conscious sedation, or whether it is performed in an operating room or a procedure suite. This distinction may be useful in separating complex procedures from simple procedures, but even this is probably mostly a reflection on traditional mind-set. For example, even thoracoscopic lobectomy is being performed under local anesthesia regularly at some centers,[21–23] and most interventional pulmonologists who are focused on this specialty are comfortable in the operating room environment and in performing procedures under anesthesia. Therefore, the distinction of the anesthetic technique and facility setting is not likely reflective of an inherent difference as much as it is of habit and tradition, and thus is not a good basis for making a distinction.

Pleuroscopy is sometimes defined as being limited to the pleura itself, whereas procedures that involve the lung are considered to be thoracoscopic. However, this distinction is also gray, considering that malignant pleural effusions and empyema often extensively involve the visceral pleura. Another distinction has been that pleuroscopy should refer to procedures in patients who do not have pleural adhesions. However, it is often difficult to reliably predict this finding before the procedure. Furthermore, what degree of adhesions is sufficient to push a procedure over the line from pleuroscopy to thoracoscopy? These considerations make it clear that both procedures examine the inside of the chest, but that existing definitions do not define clear distinctions between pleuroscopy and thoracoscopy.

FRAMING THE DISCUSSION

Those who are able to successfully complete medical school are also able to learn to function in any area of medicine. It is not a question of whether people have the ability to master a skill, but rather a question of what constitutes their training and scope of practice. Given differences in how training is structured in different parts of the world, it is also clear that there are many ways to become adequately skilled in a particular field. As medical care shifts to more of a multidisciplinary team approach within focused areas, boundaries between skills needed by different team members become less distinct. For example, cardiac anesthesiologists become adept at performing transesophageal echocardiograms and use it to assess valve function, contractility, and regional wall motion changes. In many parts of the world, pulmonologists focused on lung cancer administer chemotherapy. Boundaries are generally artificial and of our own making; it is less a matter of what could be done as it is a matter of what should be done in a particular environment.

It is crucial to recognize the importance of the setting when discussing thoracic interventional procedures. The fact that a physician working in Africa might become particularly experienced in pleural interventions to deal with tuberculous empyemas does not necessarily imply that every physician of the same specialty in another part of the world should be the person to perform this procedure. Although it is feasible to learn this procedure, as described earlier, does it make sense for the practitioner to assume the role in a different practice environment? The setting has a large impact on which is the best way to structure particular aspects of a patient's care, and includes such aspects as the size of the institution, the depth and breadth of the multidisciplinary team, and specific local needs and challenges.

An approach to the topic of invasive pleural procedures is to consider the nature of the procedure, potential risks, and ways of managing complications caused by the procedure. This approach can be used to build a framework to assess which skills and structural components should be available to those who undertake these procedures. This is a more practical approach, which allows processes for disease management to evolve without being constrained by history, preconceived attitudes, or artificial boundaries.

We must free ourselves from emotional reactions, and from assessments based on personal financial, egotistical, or professional incentives or disincentives, because these are less likely to result in approaches that stand the test of time. We should not be driven by what has been done in the past, by what can be done sometimes, or by what one can often get away with. We must learn to identify relevant inherent characteristics of the patients, diseases, and interventions, and recognize the available skills, resources, and limitations that exist in that particular institutional setting. We must use end points related to patient outcomes as the basis for constructing optimal systems of care. Although this approach is subject to challenges from people with particular viewpoints, it is more likely to persevere because the basis of the disease management is more fundamentally correct. The route taken, including type of subspecialty training, location of procedure, and type of anesthesia, matters less when the measurement is patient-centered procedural outcomes. Of course, ongoing evaluation of results achieved is necessary.

CATEGORIES OF PLEURAL PROCEDURES

Issues to consider with respect to pleural procedures include the technical difficulty of the procedure itself. Perhaps more important is the risk of either serious short-term complications (eg, major bleeding) or complications with significant long-term implications (eg, loss of function of part of the lung or diaphragm or development of a chronically infected space). The nature of potential complications is important: a complication that requires immediate attention (eg, bleeding) or expertise to avoid long-term problems necessitates a different level of backup and planning than a complication that evolves more slowly, allowing time to organize further input or even transfer of the patient to another level of care if needed. Perhaps the most difficult issue is the ability to identify cases that are potentially more challenging or risky from those that are straightforward before beginning the procedure. Associated conditions or previous history can play a major role, but some things remain more difficult to predict.

A list of pleural procedures and a qualitative assessment of important considerations are provided in **Table 1**. These procedures include some that do not typically fall under the realm of thoracoscopy, but are germane to the discussion of potential problems. A place to start the discussion is with diagnostic pleural procedures. There is little potential for acute or long-term complications when obtaining pleural biopsies in a patient with relatively normal pleura and an enigmatic effusion. Pleural nodules are still straightforward, but if there is the possibility of mesothelioma, the biopsy site should be located in a way to facilitate excision of the biopsy site (ie, along a thoracotomy incision) if curative intent resection might be considered. Such considerations are easy to learn, but familiarity with definitive management of mesothelioma may not be standard knowledge, even for thoracic surgeons.

Management of a noninfected effusion is also associated with little risk of potential acute or long-term complications, although the presence of adhesions and underlying lung disease may significantly complicate the management by adding an ongoing air leak to the initial problem of an effusion. Most often, pneumothorax is managed

Table 1
Categorization of pleural procedures

Procedure	Usual Technical Difficulty	Risk of Unanticipated More Complex Situation	Potential Complicating Factors	Potential for Major Complications		Overall Category[a]
				Acute	Chronic	
Diagnostic						
Biopsy of normal pleura (undiagnosed effusion, no nodules)	Very low	Very low	Previous procedures	Very low	Very low	CS
Biopsy of pleural nodules/masses on chest CT	Very low	Low	Adhesions	Low	Low	SF
Biopsy/pleurodesis of mesothelioma	Moderate	Moderate	Adhesions	Moderate	Moderate	CBC
Decortication/pleurectomy of mesothelioma	High	High	Comorbidities	High	High	WWIT
Therapeutic for Effusion (not Infected)						
Drainage of fluid	Very low	Very low	Previous procedures	Very low	Very low	CS
Insertion of tunneled pleural catheter	Very low	Very low	Previous procedures	Very low	Very low	CS
Talc poudrage (pleurodesis)	Very low	Very low	Previous procedures	Very low	Low	CS
Insertion of tunneled pleural catheter under direct vision	Low	Very low	Previous procedures	Very low	Very low	CS
Lysis of adhesions/destruction of loculations, pleurodesis	Low	Moderate	Previous procedures	Low	Very low	SF
Therapeutic for Effusion (Infected)						
Drainage of simple empyema (thoracentesis, tube, ± TPA)	Very low	Low	Adhesions	Very low	Very low	CS
Drainage of complex empyema (lysis of adhesions/loculations)	Low	Moderate	TB, lung disease	Very low	Very low	SF
Decortication,[b] loosely adherent	Moderate	Moderate	Comorbidities	Low	Low	CBC
Decortication,[b] densely adherent, via thoracotomy	Moderate	Moderate	Lung disease	Moderate	Low	CBC
Drainage of lung abscess and decortication	High	High	TB, lung disease	Moderate	High	WWIT
Management of chronic empyema cavity	High	High	TB, lung disease	Moderate	High	WWIT
Therapeutic for Pneumothorax						
Evacuation of pneumothorax	Very low	Low	COPD, previous events	Very low	Very low	CS
Evacuation of pneumothorax and pleurodesis	Very low	Low	COPD, previous events	Very low	Very low	CS
Resection of blebs and pleurodesis	Low	Low	COPD, previous events	Very low	Very low	SF
Lysis of adhesions/destruction of loculations, pleurodesis	Low	Moderate	COPD, previous events	Very low	Low	SF
Flication of major bullae	Moderate	Moderate	COPD, previous events	Low	High	WWIT
Treatment of chronic pleural fistula	High	High	COPD, ILD, and so forth	Low	High	WWIT

Abbreviations: COPD, chronic obstructive pulmonary disease; CT, computed tomography; ILD, interstitial lung disease; TB, tuberculosis; TPA, tissue plasminogen activator.

[a] Overall categories: CS, chip shot; SF, straightforward; CBC, could be challenging; WWIT, what was I thinking?.

[b] Stripping visceral pleural fibrin layer.

by surgeons, perhaps because the lung paren-chyma is clearly involved. However, unless there is severe underlying lung disease, the manage-ment is straightforward.

Management of an infected pleural space is more difficult. There are certainly many patients for whom a simple thoracentesis or drainage resolves the problem. For other patients, decorti-cation may be needed. This procedure carries more potential risks of serious bleeding from the pulmonary artery in the fissure, or incomplete reex-pansion of the lung, with the risk of a chronically in-fected pleural cavity (and open window or muscle flap transposition). The problem with management once simple drainage has not worked is that it has proved difficult to reliably predict preoperatively how involved a decortication procedure is going to be. Thus, it is easy to argue that decortication should be reserved for the hands of surgeons with extensive thoracic experience.

ASSESSING THE PROCESS OF PROVIDING CARE FOR PLEURAL CONDITIONS

By which measures should the level of service provided with respect to pleural procedures be judged? Obvious measures are the rate of achieving resolution of the problem at hand, and the ability to achieve this with a low rate of compli-cations. It is easier to measure this rate with respect to pleural diagnostic procedures or pneu-mothorax. Because of the varying degrees of complexity of the disease process, this process is more difficult in the case of pleural effusions, particularly when associated with infection. Was the process worse to begin with and therefore required further interventions, or did poor quality of the initial procedure (or judgment) lead to addi-tional procedures that could have been avoided?

Less obvious measures of how well pleural issues are managed are how burdensome the manage-ment is for the patient, and also for the institution and practitioners. The burden of care is a combina-tion of how long it takes until resolution, the number of days in the hospital, the amount of pain and anxiety of the patient, and other factors. A compre-hensive way to assess this situation is needed; look-ing at 1 aspect does not give the whole picture. It may be less burdensome to undergo an early thor-acoscopic drainage and partial decortication with rapid resolution than to spend days undergoing less invasive attempts (eg, chest tube, instillation of intrapleural lytics), which may have a diminished chance of success. On the other hand, this strategy is not always necessary.

The level of invasiveness is important, but of limited value in discussing the relative merits of

involvement of an interventional pulmonologist versus a thoracic surgeon. Most pleural procedures carried out by surgeons are performed by VATS in essentially every institution with any degree of thoracic surgical specialization. Decades ago, there may have been a significant difference between a thoracotomy and nonsurgical approaches; how-ever, to argue that there is a difference in invasive-ness between a surgical thoracoscopy and a medical pleuroscopy for the same patient's clinical problem borders on being ridiculous.

An important aspect of what a patient experi-ences is the system of care that exists to deliver it. This situation affects the efficiency, the extent to which outcomes and processes are critically as-sessed, and whether opportunities for improvement are identified. It may be better to enhance a system that is already in place and working well than to try to develop a new system when considering how to integrate pleuroscopy into the approach to pleural disease. The value of an existing system and how much effort it takes to create a new, well-functioning one should not be underestimated.

A critical aspect of care delivery is having a champion who is interested and takes ownership of making sure that the system of care works well. Pleural diseases are not the most glamorous, and often patients are managed because it is neces-sary but with little interest in the diseases or the overall process of care delivery. This situation is probably more true of most thoracic surgeons than interventional pulmonologists. Whatever the local situation, the value of a champion cannot be overemphasized.

DRAWING CONCLUSIONS

How do we deliver the best care for patients with pleural conditions? How does this discussion help us integrate thoracoscopy, pleuroscopy, and other pleural procedures into an efficient, high-quality, programmatic approach?

It is clear that some pleural conditions are more straightforward and lend themselves more easily to being managed by practitioners with a variety of backgrounds, if they have the interest and acquire the necessary skills. Others, such as management of more complex pleural infections, require more experience and judgment.

It is also clear that how care is delivered depends on many different factors in a particular institution, and there is no simple answer that fits all situations. It depends on local availability of expertise from various individuals, constraints on people's time, and the ability to deliver care in various settings (ie, the operating room vs proce-dure suite; the use of general anesthesia vs conscious sedation). The value of a dedicated interest in organizing the care process and proactively working to make it better is crucial.

It is also clear that exceptional care requires a team that works together seamlessly. No matter how focused, experienced or knowledgeable any individual is, there are always limits. As medical knowledge progresses, and there is an ever greater amount of literature and skills to be mastered, we must transform from individual practitioners delivering care to care delivered by individuals who function collaboratively within a team. This approach allows collective knowledge, judgment, and skills to be applied to the problem at hand.

It does not benefit us to argue about semantics, backgrounds of a practitioner, or how access to the pleural space is attained. Time is better spent reviewing results of the pleural procedure to ensure that the process of care delivery optimizes the results for the patient and the care system. As we provide thoracoscopic care in 2013 and beyond, it behooves us to define that care more in terms of appropriate access to the pleural space, with the anticipated results and minimal complications, than to maintain useless definitions based on who performed the procedure and where.

REFERENCES

1. Shigemura N, Akashi A, Funaki S, et al. Long-term outcomes after a variety of video-assisted thoracoscopic lobectomy approaches for clinical stage IA lung cancer: a multi-institutional study. J Thorac Cardiovasc Surg 2006;132(3):507–12.
2. Swanson SJ, Herndon JE II, D'Amico TA, et al. Video-assisted thoracic surgery lobectomy: report of CALGB 39802 a prospective, multi-institution feasibility study. J Clin Oncol 2007;25(31):4993–7.
3. Rocco G, Internullo E, Cassivi S, et al. The variability of practice in minimally invasive thoracic surgery for pulmonary resections. Thorac Surg Clin 2008;18(3):235–47.
4. Roviaro G, Rebuffat C, Varoli F, et al. Videoendoscopic pulmonary lobectomy for cancer. Surg Laparosc Endosc 1992;2(3):244–7.
5. Cheng D, Downey RJ, Kernstine K, et al. Video-assisted thoracic surgery in lung cancer resection: a meta-analysis and systematic review of controlled trials. Innovations 2007;2(6):261–92.
6. Detterbeck F. Thoracoscopic vs. open lobectomy debate: the pro argument. Thorac Surg Sci 2009;6:1–9.
7. Whitson BA, Groth SS, Duval SJ, et al. Surgery for early-stage non-small cell lung cancer: a systematic review of the video-assisted thoracoscopic surgery versus thoracotomy approaches to lobectomy. Ann Thorac Surg 2008;86(6):2008–18.
8. Yan TD, Black D, Bannon PG, et al. Systematic review and meta-analysis of randomized and nonrandomized trials on safety and efficacy of video-assisted thoracic surgery lobectomy for early-stage non-small-cell lung cancer. J Clin Oncol 2009;27(15):2553–62.
9. Demmy TL, Nwogu C. Is video-assisted thoracic surgery lobectomy better? Quality of life considerations. Ann Thorac Surg 2008;85(2):S719–28.
10. McKenna RJ Jr, Houck W, Fuller CB. Video-assisted thoracic surgery lobectomy: experience with 1,100 cases. Ann Thorac Surg 2006;81:421–6.
11. Park H, Detterbeck F, Boffa D, et al. Impact of hospital volume of thoracoscopic lobectomy on primary lung cancer outcomes. Ann Thorac Surg 2012;93(2):372–9.
12. Paul S, Altorki NK, Sheng S, et al. Thoracoscopic lobectomy is associated with lower morbidity than open lobectomy: a propensity-matched analysis from the STS database. J Thorac Cardiovasc Surg 2010;139(2):366–78.
13. Craig SR, Leaver HA, Yap PL, et al. Acute phase responses following minimal access and conventional thoracic surgery. Eur J Cardiothorac Surg 2001;20(3):455–63.
14. Kirby TJ, Mack MJ, Landreneau RJ, et al. Lobectomy–video-assisted thoracic surgery versus muscle-sparing thoracotomy: a randomized trial. J Thorac Cardiovasc Surg 1995;109:997–1002.
15. Sugi K, Kaneda Y, Esato K. Video-assisted thoracoscopic lobectomy achieves a satisfactory long-term prognosis in patients with clinical stage IA lung cancer. World J Surg 2000;24(1):27–31.
16. Boffa DJ, Allen MS, Grab JD, et al. Data from the society of thoracic surgeons general thoracic surgery database: the surgical management of primary lung tumors. J Thorac Cardiovasc Surg 2008;135(2):247–54.
17. Tovar E. Minimally invasive approach for pneumonectomy culminating in an outpatient procedure. Chest 1998;114:1454–8.
18. Nwogu CE, Glinianski M, Demmy TL. Minimally invasive pneumonectomy. Ann Thorac Surg 2006;82(1):e3–4.
19. D'Amico TA. Thoracoscopic segmentectomy: technical considerations and outcomes. Ann Thorac Surg 2008;85(2):S716–8.
20. Mahtabifard A, Fuller CB, McKenna RJ Jr. Video-assisted thoracic surgery sleeve lobectomy: a case series. Ann Thorac Surg 2008;85(2):S729–32.
21. Rocco G, Romano V, Accardo R, et al. Awake single-access (Uniportal) video-assisted thoracoscopic surgery for peripheral pulmonary nodules in a complete ambulatory setting. Ann Thorac Surg 2010;89(5):1625–7.
22. Pompeo E, Mineo TC. Awake operative videothoracoscopic pulmonary resections. Thorac Surg Clin 2008;18(3):311–20.
23. Pompeo E. Awake thoracic surgery–is it worth the trouble? Semin Thorac Cardiovasc Surg 2012;24(2):106–14.

Malignant Pleural Mesothelioma
Update on Treatment Options with a Focus on Novel Therapies

Andrew R. Haas, MD, PhD, Daniel H. Sterman, MD*

KEYWORDS

- Malignant pleural mesothelioma • Radiation therapy • Chemotherapy • Multimodal therapy
- Gene therapy

KEY POINTS

- In the past decade, advances have been made that have improved the ability to treat malignant pleural mesothelioma.
- There is evidence that these treatments are increasing the quality and quantity of life for patients with mesothelioma.
- Multimodality treatment programs that combine maximal surgical cytoreduction with novel forms of radiation therapy and more effective chemotherapy combinations may offer significant increases in survival for certain subgroups of patients with mesothelioma.
- Lung-sparing surgery may allow improvements in pulmonary function after surgery-based multimodality therapy, and potential longer overall survival than that seen with extrapleural pneumonectomy.
- Experimental treatments such as immunotherapy and gene therapy provide hope for all patients with mesothelioma, and in the future may be combined with standard therapy in multimodality protocols.

Mesothelioma is an insidious mesothelial neoplasm originating in the pleura, pericardium, peritoneum, or tunica vaginalis, with approximately 80% of cases involving the thorax. The predominant cause of malignant mesothelioma is exposure to asbestos. The incidence of mesothelioma in the United States is estimated to be approximately 2000 to 3000 cases per year, with an increasing incidence worldwide, secondary to the proliferation and poor regulation of industrial and household use of asbestos.[1–6]

A nihilistic attitude regarding mesothelioma has persisted among many physicians because of significant associated morbidity and mortality, as well as poor response to standard therapeutic interventions. However, novel treatment paradigms offer hope for enhanced palliation, improved tumor responses, and prolonged survival.[6–9] This article focuses on standard therapeutic interventions for malignant pleural mesothelioma (MPM) such as surgery, chemotherapy, and radiation therapy, as well as experimental approaches such as targeted therapy, immunotherapy, and gene-based therapies.

SURGERY FOR MPM

Surgery for MPM can be diagnostic, palliative, or cytoreductive, although it is potentially associated with significant morbidity and mortality. The

Section of Interventional Pulmonology and Thoracic Oncology, Pulmonary, Allergy, and Critical Care Division, University of Pennsylvania Medical Center, 833 West Gates Building, 3400 Spruce Street, Philadelphia, PA 19104-4283, USA
* Corresponding author.
E-mail address: daniel.sterman@uphs.upenn.edu

Clin Chest Med 34 (2013) 99–111
http://dx.doi.org/10.1016/j.ccm.2012.12.005
0272-5231/13/$ – see front matter © 2013 Elsevier Inc. All rights reserved.

chestmed.theclinics.com

development of thoracoscopy has allowed earlier diagnosis of mesothelioma. However, most patients with MPM have advanced disease at diagnosis, as well as comorbid medical illnesses, which often precludes aggressive surgical intervention.

Dyspnea from the accumulation of a pleural effusion is the most common presenting symptom of MPM. For symptomatic effusions in MPM, the optimal palliative approach is maximal drainage of the effusion and subsequent pleurodesis. The most widely used compound for pleurodesis in MPM is sterile talc, administered either as a powder (poudrage) via thoracoscopy or as a slurry via tube thoracostomy.[10] The presence of bulky tumor in the pleural space, or entrapment of the lung by a thick visceral pleural peel, is a contraindication to pleurodesis in patients with MPM. Attempts at talc pleurodesis in the setting of lung entrapment can lead to a multiloculated pleural space with a high risk of empyema. In this setting of lung entrapment in MPM, the preferred intervention is insertion of a tunneled intrapleural catheter to drain recurrent effusions and provide effective palliation of dyspnea (**Fig. 1**).[11] The primary concern regarding the use of tunneled pleural catheters (TPCs) in mesothelioma is the development of tumor implants at the insertion site or along the subcutaneous tunnel.[11,12] Recent reports of TPCs for malignant pleural effusions (MPEs) show equivalent results for the control of effusions compared with talc slurry pleurodesis. Therefore, TPCs should be considered for management of symptomatic effusions in patients with MPM, even in those whose lungs are unable to expand.[13] Pleuroperiotoneal shunting, an alternative approach for dealing with lung entrapment in pleural mesothelioma, carries the overt risk of malignant seeding of the peritoneal cavity, and is therefore infrequently used.

Thoracoscopic parietal pleurectomy is an alternative to talc pleurodesis in reducing the recurrence of pleural effusions in mesothelioma, and with less morbidity than open pleurectomy.[14] Complete parietal and visceral pleurectomy (pleurectomy/decortication) may palliate dyspnea in patients with mesothelioma with bulky intrapleural disease with or without lung entrapment, but by itself has not been shown to prolong survival.[15]

Extrapleural pneumonectomy (EPP) is en bloc resection of the lung, the parietal and visceral pleurae, and portions of the ipsilateral pericardium and diaphragm. It provides maximal tumor cytoreduction and facilitates higher radiation dosage to the involved hemithorax. EPP alone has no influence on survival in the absence of adjuvant therapy. In most surgical series of EPP in MPM, median survival is less than 2 years, with average 5-year survival rates of 10% to 20%.[15–18] However, there are long-term survivors following EPP for maximal cytoreduction as a component of multimodality treatment involving adjuvant radiation therapy and postoperative chemotherapy.[19–21] However, the benefits of EPP with adjuvant chemotherapy with or without local radiotherapy are limited to otherwise healthy patients with early-stage disease, epithelial histology, and no mediastinal lymph node involvement. Patients with biphasic or sarcomatoid histology and/or mediastinal or hilar node positivity have an ominous prognosis.[19]

Several approaches for adjuvant therapy in conjunction with EPP have been studied. Investigators at Brigham and Women's Hospital in Boston

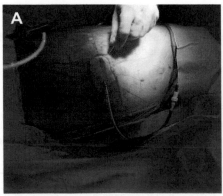
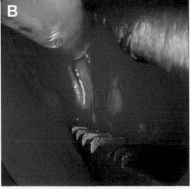

Fig. 1. (*A*) Tunneled pleural catheters (TPCs) are an important method of palliation in patients with mesothelioma and recurrent symptomatic pleural effusions. (*B*) Thoracoscopic placement of TPCs can be performed even in the setting of prior talc pleurodesis to facilitate intrapleural instillation of experimental therapies. (*Courtesy of* Dr Joseph Friedberg, Division of Thoracic Surgery, Perelman School of Medicine of the University of Pennsylvania, Philadelphia, PA.)

initially combined EPP with sequential postoperative chemotherapy and adjuvant external beam radiation therapy to the ipsilateral hemithorax.[19–21] More recently, the Brigham group has investigated the role of hyperthermic intracavitary chemotherapy as an adjuvant to maximal cytoreductive surgery, in combination with hemithoracic irradiation and systemic chemotherapy.[22,23] Other novel multicenter clinical trials combine maximal surgical debulking with adjuvant intensity-modulated radiation therapy (IMRT), or alternatively assess the role of neoadjuvant chemotherapy before cytoreductive surgery to improve long-term outcomes.[24]

Other investigators have evaluated the usefulness of postresectional photodynamic therapy (PDT) (**Fig. 2**). The single randomized trial of this technology in MPM, conducted by Pass and colleagues[25] at the National Cancer Institute in the early 1990s, failed to confirm any benefit for adjuvant PDT compared with surgery alone with or without adjuvant chemotherapy/immunotherapy. More recent data by Friedberg and colleagues[26,27] showed improvements in overall survival compared with historical controls and improved outcomes with PDT after radical pleurectomy compared with outcomes after EPP. Novel photosensitizers are currently under study that may provide better local control, decreased photosensitivity, and perhaps improved induction of systemic antitumor immune responses.

There have been several recent promising reports about the use of radical pleurectomy as a maximal debulking procedure in multimodality protocols (**Fig. 3**), with various adjuvant intraoperative therapies such as intrapleural PDT, intrapleural hyperthermic chemotherapy (cisplatin, gemcitabine), and hyperthermic perfusion with povidone-iodine,[27,28] which have also been administered in association with IMRT in the presence of intact lung with demonstration of preserved/improved pulmonary function.[29]

RADIATION THERAPY FOR MPM

Contrary to the prevailing wisdom that MPM is a radioresistant neoplasm, mesothelioma cell lines in vitro may be more responsive to ionizing radiation than non–small cell lung cancer cell lines. However, external beam radiation therapy for mesothelioma is limited by the large treatment volumes required and the radiation sensitivity of the surrounding organs (heart, lung, esophagus, spinal cord).

Although palliative radiotherapy with an attempt to treat the entire involved pleural surface is technically difficult and associated with a high risk of radiation pneumonitis, myelitis, hepatitis, and myocarditis, it can provide effective local palliation in up to 50% of patients.[30] There are also anecdotal reports of long-term survivors following high-dose external beam irradiation and even intrapleural administration of radioactive isotopes.[30] Furthermore, radiation therapy may play a role by preventing chest wall recurrences after thoracoscopy/thoracotomy and in improving local control after pleurectomy or extrapleural pneumonectomy. Mesothelioma frequently implants along the tracts of biopsies, chest tubes, thoracoscopy trocars, and surgical incisions, producing uncomfortable subcutaneous nodules. This outcome can be prevented with prophylactic radiotherapy. In a small randomized trial, Boutin and colleagues[31] showed that 21 Gy administered in 3 daily fractions, 10 to 15 days after thoracoscopy, significantly decreased local recurrence at incision sites. These findings have been confirmed by other investigators.[32–34]

Multimodality approaches commonly include adjuvant radiation following surgery, although there are no randomized trials that show its efficacy. Because the lung remains in place after pleurectomy, radiotherapy doses must be lower than when EPP is performed.[30]

The Radiation Oncology group at the University of Texas MD Anderson Cancer Center reported encouraging results using IMRT following EPP. Using careful treatment planning and IMRT, radiation doses of up to 50 to 60 Gy were possible without severe toxicity. With the combination of EPP and IMRT, local recurrences after surgery were virtually eliminated; however, novel distant disease patterns have begun to emerge. These

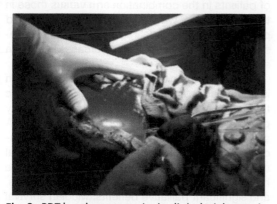

Fig. 2. PDT has shown promise in clinical trials as an intraoperative adjunctive therapy after maximal cytoreductive surgery. PDT can improve local control by direct cell killing of microscopic residual disease in the postoperative hemithorax as well as inducing systemic antitumor responses that may result in prolongation of median survival. (*Courtesy of* Dr Joseph Friedberg, Division of Thoracic Surgery, Perelman School of Medicine of the University of Pennsylvania, Philadelphia, PA.)

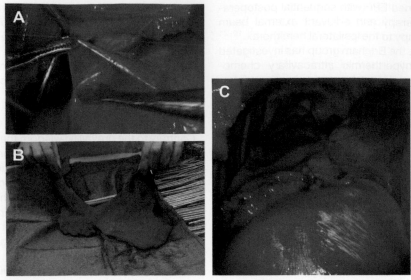

Fig. 3. Radical pleurectomy as a lung-sparing modality of maximal surgical debulking in MPM. (*A*) Dissection of visceral pleura off the surface of a lung. (*B*) Radical pleurectomy specimen in patient with early-stage mesothelioma. (*C*) Right lower lobe after completion of radical pleurectomy with full reexpansion. (*Courtesy of Dr Joseph Friedberg, Division of Thoracic Surgery, Perelman School of Medicine of the University of Pennsylvania, Philadelphia, PA.*)

data suggest that the combination of EPP and IMRT requires an additional treatment modality (ie, chemotherapy or immunotherapy) to limit distant tumor growth. Although IMRT following EPP seemed to be more effective for local disease control in this initial series, a second series suggested that there was a significant increase in severe toxicity (6 of 13 patients developed fatal pneumonitis).[35] More recent studies have shown the safety of IMRT in MPM, even in the presence of an intact lung in the adjuvant setting.[24,29] Novel forms of radiation therapy, including proton beam therapy, are currently under investigation for treatment of MPM.

CHEMOTHERAPY FOR MPM

The current standard of care for first-line systemic therapy in patients with unresectable MPM with good performance status is combination chemotherapy with pemetrexed and cisplatin. Pemetrexed (Alimta, Eli Lilly and Company, Indianapolis, IN) is a multitargeted antifolate compound that blocks several enzymes in the folate metabolism pathway. Pemetrexed is a potent inhibitor of thymidylate synthase (TS), the rate-limiting enzyme in the synthesis of thymidylate, which is required for DNA synthesis. TS is also the enzyme inhibited by the cytotoxic agents 5-fluorouracil and raltitrexed.[9,36]

In 2003, Vogelzang and colleagues[9] reported the results of a phase III randomized clinical trial in 456 chemotherapy-naive patients with MPM comparing treatment with pemetrexed and cisplatin with cisplatin monotherapy. Response rates were 41.3% in the pemetrexed/cisplatin arm versus 16.7% in the control arm ($P<.0001$). Median time to progression was significantly longer in the pemetrexed/cisplatin arm: 5.7 months versus 3.9 months ($P = .001$). Median survival time in the pemetrexed/cisplatin arm was 12.1 months versus 9.3 months in the cisplatin-only arm ($P = .020$, 2-sided log-rank test). The hazard ratio for death of patients in the combination arm versus those in the control arm was 0.77. Another randomized phase III study of cisplatin and raltitrexed in unresectable MPM showed similar increases in median survival.[37]

The combination of gemcitabine and carboplatin is also an acceptable first-line option for systemic therapy for MPM because of its acceptable toxicity profile, good response rate, and palliative effects. A single-arm, northern Italian, phase II study of gemcitabine and carboplatin in patients with pleural mesothelioma reported a 26% partial response rate, a median response duration of 55 weeks, and significant palliative benefits. Median survival for patients in this study was 66 weeks.[38–40] A recent randomized clinical trial showed no benefit from the addition of bevacizumab to this regimen.[41]

However, there is no current standard of care for second-line chemotherapy in mesothelioma following treatment with cisplatin and pemetrexed. The most commonly used second-line regimens include gemcitabine or other drugs with single-agent activity such as vinorelbine. There exists insufficient evidence to recommend second-line chemotherapy as a standard treatment. Patients with adequate performance status should be enrolled into clinical trials of second-line treatment.[42–46] A large, double-blinded, randomized clinical trial of the histone deacetylase inhibitor vorinistat in second-line therapy for MPM showed no survival benefit for the study drug compared with placebo.[47]

TARGETED THERAPY

The presence of active platelet-derived growth factor (PDGF) and epidermal growth factor (EGF) pathways in some mesothelioma cell lines in vitro implied that novel inhibitors of these pathways might prove useful clinically, either as monotherapy or in combination with chemotherapy. However, early-phase clinical trials of imatinib mesylate and gefitinib (and erlotinib), inhibitors of the tyrosine kinases critical to the PDGF and EGF pathways respectively, failed to show any significant clinical benefits in MPM.[48–51] Clinical trials were conducted with other novel targeted agents, such as the antiangiogenic agents, bevacizumab and thalidomide, and the copper-chelating agent, tetrathiomolybdate, which depletes copper, a key cofactor in tumor angiogenesis. Only the tetrathiomolybdate has shown any benefit in human trials.[25,52,53]

NEW THERAPEUTIC APPROACHES

Despite the improvements in survival achieved with surgery-based multimodality therapy and combination chemotherapy for MPM, less morbid, more effective interventions are needed. Addressing the focality of the disease process within the involved hemithorax, many investigators have attempted to treat MPM by direct instillation of chemotherapeutic and other therapeutic agents into the pleural space, but without much success.[54–56] Based on case reports of spontaneous tumor remissions and associations of intratumoral lymphocytic infiltration with improved median survival rates, several groups have investigated immunotherapeutic approaches for MPM as a potential means of achieving better tumor response rates.[2]

IMMUNOTHERAPY

The use of compounds to stimulate an antitumor immune response against pleural malignancy stemmed from the observation that patients who developed postoperative empyemas after lung cancer resection had improved survival rates.[57–59]

Intrapleural bacille Calmette-Guérin (BCG) was subsequently studied as a surgical adjuvant, but no significant clinical benefits were noted.[60] Several systemic immunotherapies have been administered to patients with MPM, including interleukin (IL)-2 and interferon gamma (IFN-γ), both of which showed limited efficacy and significant side effects. Subcutaneous IFN-α-2a was found to be partially efficacious and reasonably well tolerated, with a 14% overall response rate as monotherapy for MPM.[61] One European phase I to II study of intrapleural IL-2 administered by continuous infusion via an indwelling catheter revealed a 19% partial response rate, but with marked dose-related toxicity, primarily the development of empyemas.[62]

Boutin and colleagues[63,64] in Marseilles, France, pioneered the intrapleural administration of immunostimulatory cytokines to treat MPM, showing significant local tumor responses with both intrapleural IL-2 and IFN-γ. Most impressive were the results of intrapleural IFN-γ in patients with early-stage mesothelioma (tumor localized to the parietal ± visceral pleural surfaces), with an overall response rate of 20%. Furthermore, 17 of 89 patients treated had histologically confirmed partial or complete responses on follow-up thoracoscopy. Overall, patients with stage I disease had a response rate of 45%.

Other groups showed only limited activity with intrapleural IL-2, and with the combination of intrapleural IFN-γ and autologous activated macrophages. Immunotherapy trials in Australia showed some significant tumor regression with repeated intratumoral injection of granulocyte-monocyte colony-stimulating factor (GM-CSF), but with complications related to the catheters used for cytokine instillation.[65–67]

GENE THERAPY

In the absence of curative therapies for MPM, several groups have investigated the nascent technologies of gene transfer as a potential mediator of antitumor responses in MPM (**Table 1**).[68] Intrapleural gene therapy for mesothelioma is attractive because the disease typically remains localized for most of its course, and access to the tumor in the pleural cavity is easy and safe. Gene transfer delivery systems (vectors) used in preclinical and clinical studies were either liposomal/DNA complexes or modified viruses, including herpes, vaccinia, and adenoviruses. Therapeutic genes delivered by these vectors included so-called suicide genes, cytokines, tumor suppressor genes (ie, p53), and proapoptotic genes. Studies have also been conducted using replication-restricted,

Table 1
Intrapleural gene therapy trials for mesothelioma

Study	Phase	Histology	Total No. (# Evaluable)	Agent	Delivery	Best Clinical Response	Additional Outcome Measures
Sterman et al,[72] 1998	I	MPM	21	Ad.HSVtk/GCV	Intrapleural: single dose; GCV × 14 d	Gene transfer confirmed in 11 of 20 evaluable patients in a dose-related fashion	Strong antiadenoviral immune responses generated, including high titers of neutralizing antibody and T-cell proliferative responses
Sterman et al,[73] 2000	I	MPM	8	Ad.HSVtk/GCV + corticosteroids	Intrapleural: single dose; GCV × 14 d	Two long-term survivors with stable disease for 6 y after treatment	Safety and toxicity without difference from initial clinical trial
Sterman et al,[80] 2007	I	MPM MPE	MPM: 7 MPE: 3	Ad.IFN-β	Intrapleural: single dose	1 (10%) with CR, 2 (20%) with PR, 4 (40%) with SD	Successful gene transfer, induction of humoral/innate immune response
Dong, 2008[84]	I	MM MPE	Treatment = 27; Control = 21	Ad.wt-p53 ± IP cisplatin	Intrapleural/intraperitoneal: weekly × 4	Total effective rates for the treatment group (63.0%) and for the control group (42.9%)	Safety and toxicity
Sterman et al,[81] 2010	I	MPM MPE	MPM: 10 MPE: 7	Ad.IFN-β	Intrapleural: 2 doses	3 (18%) with PR/MR 11 (61%) with SD	Successful gene transfer with first dose but not second, induction of humoral immune response

Sterman et al,[82] 2011	I	MPM	9	Ad.IFN-α-2b	Intrapleural: 2 doses	2 (22%) PR, 4 (44%) with SD	Ad.IFN-α induced much higher levels of gene transfer than Ad.INFβ. Induction of humoral/innate immune response
Schwarzenberger et al,[76] 2011	I	MPM	15	PA1-STK cells/GCV	Multiple intrapleural infusion (every 4 wk × 3) followed by 7 d of intravenous GCV	CR (0%), PR (0%) and stable disease (9%) and (3%) at 3 and 6 mo, respectively	Median overall survival from the time of treatment initiation: 7.7 mo
Sterman/Haas, 2012	IIA	MPM	Ongoing	Ad.IFN-α-2b	Intrapleural: 2 doses with: 1. Pemetrexed + platin 2. Gemcitabine ± platin	Ongoing	Gene transfer, immune response, safety, and toxicity

Abbreviations: Ad, adenovirus; Ad.wt-p53, adenovirus wild-type p53 gene construct; CR, complete response; DCC-E1A, liposomal E1A gene conjugate; IFN-α, interferon alfa; IFN-β, interferon beta; IHC, immunohistochemical staining; MPE, malignant pleural effusion; MPM, malignant pleural mesothelioma; MR, mixed response; PD, progressive disease; PR, partial response; RT-PCR, reverse transcriptase-polymerase chain reaction; SD, stable disease.

tumor-selective adenoviruses and herpes viruses, as well as carrier cells, such as modified ovarian carcinoma cells (OVCAR-3).[68,69]

CLINICAL INVESTIGATIONS OF GENE THERAPY IN MPM
Suicide Gene Therapy

Suicide gene therapy involves transduction of tumor cells with a gene encoding an enzyme that induces sensitivity to an otherwise benign therapeutic agent. In essence, a prodrug is transformed into a toxic metabolite by introduction of the enzyme into the malignant cells with subsequent accumulation leading to tumor cell death or suicide.[70,71] A major advantage of suicide gene therapy is the induction of a bystander effect; the killing of neighboring cells not transduced with the vector. A commonly studied suicide gene is the herpes simplex virus-1 thymidine kinase (HSVtk) gene, which makes transduced cells sensitive to the nucleoside analogue ganciclovir (GCV). GCV is metabolized poorly by mammalian cells and thus is usually nontoxic. However, after conversion to GCV-monophosphate by HSVtk, it is metabolized rapidly by endogenous kinases to GCV-triphosphate, which acts as a potent inhibitor of DNA polymerase and competes with normal mammalian nucleosides for DNA replication.[70,71]

Based on data from extensive preclinical studies, our group at the University of Pennsylvania in 1995 initiated a series of phase 1 clinical trials of adenoviral suicide gene therapy (Ad.HSVtk/GCV) in patients with advanced MPM to assess toxicity, gene transfer efficiency, and immune response induction.[72–74] After a single intrapleural administration of Ad.HSVtk vector, GCV was given intravenously twice daily for 2 weeks. Dose-related intratumoral HSVtk gene transfer was shown in 23 of 30 patients, with those treated at a dose greater than or equal to 3.2×10^{11} plaque forming units (pfu) with evidence of HSVtk protein expression up to 30 to 50 cell layers deep by immunohistochemical assessment. Overall, the suicide gene therapy was well tolerated with minimal side effects and no dose-limiting toxicity. Antitumor and antiadenoviral vector immune responses, including induction of high titers of antiadenoviral neutralizing antibody and proliferative T-cell responses, were generated in both serum and pleural fluid. Several clinical responses were seen at the higher dose levels, with 2 patients showing long periods of survival (1 surviving 7 years and 1 still alive after 14 years). One of the two surviving patients had demonstrable reduction of tumor metabolic activity as assessed by serial 18-fluorodeoxyglucose (^{18}FDG) positron emission tomography (PET) scans

over several months. This long response period was hypothesized to be caused by induction of a secondary immune bystander effect of the Ad.HSVtk/GCV instillation.[72–74]

Schwarzenberger and colleagues[75,76] at Louisiana State University conducted a phase 1 trial using irradiated ovarian carcinoma cells (OVCAR-3) retrovirally transfected with HSVtk (PA1-STK cells) that were instilled intrapleurally followed by GCV for 7 days. Minimal side effects were seen, although there were some posttreatment increases in the percentage of CD8$^+$ T lymphocytes in the pleural fluid. However, no significant clinical responses were documented.

Cytokine Gene Therapy

The rationale for cytokine gene therapy is that high-level expression of immunostimulatory cytokines (such as IL-2, IL-12, tumor necrosis factor, GM-CSF, or interferons) from tumor cells activates the immune system in situ, resulting in a more effective antitumor immune response without having to target specific antigens. The advantages of cytokine gene delivery compared with systemic administration of these agents included lower toxicity, higher local concentrations, and longer persistence of the cytokine.[68]

Robinson and colleagues[69] conducted the first clinical trial of intratumoral cytokine gene delivery in patients with MPM using a replication-restricted vaccinia virus (VV) expressing the human IL-2 gene. Serial VV-IL-2 vector injections over a period of 12 weeks into chest wall lesions of 6 patients with advanced MPM resulted in minimal toxicity, but no significant tumor regression. Modest intratumoral T-cell infiltration was detected on posttreatment biopsy specimens. VV-IL-2 mRNA was detected in biopsy specimens for up to 6 days after injection despite the generation of significant levels of anti-VV–neutralizing antibodies.[77]

Based on the success of in vivo experiments,[78,79] our group at the Hospital of the University of Pennsylvania conducted the first human trial of intrapleural interferon gene therapy for MPM and MPE.[80] The study evaluated the safety and feasibility of a single-dose intrapleural IFN-β gene transfer using an adenoviral vector (Ad.IFN-β) in patients with MPM and MPE. Ad.IFN-β was administered via an indwelling pleural catheter in escalating doses in 2 cohorts of patients: MPM (7 patients) and MPE (3 patients). Subjects were evaluated for toxicity, gene transfer, immune responses, and antitumor responses via ^{18}FDG PET scans and chest computed tomography (CT) scans. Intrapleural Ad.IFN-β was well tolerated with transient lymphopenia as the most common side effect. Other side effects included hypoxia and liver function abnormalities. Gene transfer was documented in 7 of the 10 patients by demonstration of IFN-β mRNA or protein expression in pleural fluid. Antitumor immune responses were shown in 7 of the 10 patients and included the detection of cytotoxic T cells, activation of circulating natural killer cells, and humoral responses to known tumor-associated antigens as well as to allogenic mesothelioma cell lines. Four of 10 patients showed meaningful clinical responses defined as disease stability and/or regression on PET and CT scans at day 60 after vector instillation.[80] This study showed that administration of intrapleural Ad.IFN-β was feasible and well tolerated, and resulted in successful gene transfer. The study also showed that a single intrapleural dose of IFN-β vector induced demonstrable antitumor immune responses as well as anecdotal clinical responses in a heavily pretreated population of patients with MPM [80]

A second phase I trial was then conducted to determine whether using 2 doses of Ad.IFN-β vector would prove superior to a single dose.[81] Ten patients with MPM and 7 with MPE received 2 doses of Ad.IFN-β through an indwelling pleural catheter. Repeated doses were generally well tolerated. The most common adverse events were lymphopenia, hypoalbuminemia, hypotension, anemia, hypocalcemia, and mild cytokine release syndrome (CRS). One patient developed pericardial tamponade but pericardial fluid analysis did not reveal tumor cells or increased IFN-β levels.[81]

In this repeat-dose gene transfer study, high levels of IFN-β were detected in pleural fluid after the first dose; however, absent intrapleural IFN-β expression after the second dose correlated with the rapid induction of neutralizing Ad antibodies (Nabs). Antibody responses against tumor antigens were induced in most patients. At 2-month follow-up imaging, 1 patient with MPM had a partial response, 2 had stable disease, and 9 had progressive disease. On PET scanning, 2 patients had mixed responses and 11 had stable disease. There were 7 patients with survival times longer than 18 months. Overall, repeated intrapleural instillation of Ad.IFN-β vector was safe, induced immune responses, and there was some evidence of clinical responses. However, rapid development of Nabs prevented effective gene transfer after the second dose, even with a shortened dose interval of 7 days.[81]

We then designed another phase I trial to evaluate a shortened dosing interval by administering a second dose of intrapleural Ad-IFN vector 3 days after the first dose, before the expected peak of Nab production.[82] For this trial, our group used a recombinant, replication-incompetent adenovirus vector expressing the human interferon alfa-2b gene (Ad.IFN-α2b) obtained from Schering-Plough/Merck (SCH721015). Ad.IFN-α2b was instilled on study days 1 and 4 via a tunneled pleural catheter. The starting vector dose was 1×10^{12} viral particles, but this dose was reduced to 3×10^{11} after the first 3 patients developed significant CRS symptoms. Subjects were assessed for antitumor responses at day 60 using CT and PET scans. Pleural fluid and serum IFN-α2b levels, mesothelin-related protein (SMRP) levels, and Nabs were measured. In general, although most patients developed some CRS symptoms, Ad.IFN-α2b vector instillation was well tolerated. Increased and sustained serum IFN-α levels were occasionally associated with protracted flulike symptoms lasting 1 to 2 weeks. Pleural catheter-related infections occurred in 2 patients and both were treated successfully with antibiotics. Successful gene transfer and high IFN-α levels in pleural fluid were shown even in patients who received a lower dose of vector. Furthermore, there was evidence that the second Ad.IFN-α2b dose resulted in successful gene transfer. There were encouraging immunologic responses, such as new or increased intensity bands on immunoblots containing extracts of mesothelioma cell lines, in 7 of 8 patients, as well as upregulation of the activation marker CD69 on circulating natural killer cells.[82]

At initial radiographic assessment using modified Response Evaluation Criteria in Solid Tumors (RECIST) on day 60, 3 subjects had progressive disease, 4 had stable disease, and 2 had partial responses. Two patients had sufficient improvement that they were subsequently able to undergo successful radical pleurectomy, with no signs of recurrence 21 and 33 months after surgery. One patient, who has previously been treated with radical pleurectomy and chemotherapy, had an impressive radiographic and metabolic tumor response in that many of the pleural-based malignant foci had regressed on PET/CT by 2 months after vector instillations. On 6-month follow-up PET/CT after Ad.IFN-α2b, many lesions had completely resolved, most at sites distant from vector instillation. The crucial result of the study was the recognition of low levels of Nabs at the shortened dosing interval with prolonged intrapleural interferon expression.[82] The combination of a better dosing strategy as described earlier, as well as the higher potency and sustained levels of IFN-α, may result in better antitumor response in future clinical trials.

Thus, although these strategies seem to be successful in initiating antitumor immune responses,

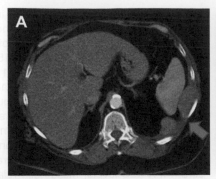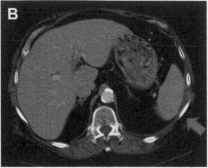

Fig. 4. (*A*) Chest CT scan of a patient newly diagnosed with biphasic mesothelioma involving the left pleural space and extending through the left chest wall and left hemidiaphragm. (*B*) Chest CT scan status post 2 weeks of high-dose COX-2 inhibitor (celecoxib) and 2 doses of intrapleural Ad.IFN-α2b vector and 4 cycles of combination chemotherapy with pemetrexed and cisplatin. Near-complete response of intrathoracic and chest wall tumor is shown (*arrowheads*).

they are limited by large tumor volumes and significant immunoinhibitory networks, even beyond Nabs. These networks, created by the tumors, involve cytokines such as TGF-β, IL-10, prostaglandin E2, vascular endothelial cell growth factor, and additionally by inhibitor cells such as T-regulatory cells and myeloid-derived suppressor cells. Ongoing clinical trials with the Ad.IFN-α2b vector involve combination with front-line and second-line chemotherapy, as well as a brief course of high-dose cyclooxygenase-2 (COX-2) inhibitor (celecoxib) for modification of the tumor microenvironment and these inhibitory networks (**Fig. 4**). Future trials are going to likely require combination approaches that stimulate the immune system, reduce tumor burden (surgery and/or chemotherapy), and inhibit the inhibitors (with agents such as COX-2 inhibitors or anti–TGF-β antibodies).

Another major approach is to use adoptive transfer of gene-modified autologous lymphocytes that have been altered ex vivo by using retroviruses or lentiviruses to augment their ability to attack mesothelioma cells, which can be done by transfection of T-cell receptors with altered specificity or by the introduction of artificial chimeric T-cell antigen receptors (CARs) that use single-chain antibody fragments to define antigen specificity and intracellular fragments of both the T-cell receptor and accessory molecules (such as CD28 or 4–1BB) to enhance activation.[83] Our group at Penn, and others at Memorial Sloan Kettering Cancer Center and the National Cancer Institute, are designing CARs to target T cells to the tumor antigen mesothelin for use in the treatment of mesothelioma. The approach has worked well in preclinical models,[83] and clinical trials using this approach have been initiated at several centers in the past 2 years.

Novel treatments such as gene therapy for MPM have not yet reached routine clinical practice. An appropriate analogy may be the development of monoclonal antibodies, which took more than 20 years from discovery to clinical application. Despite what some perceive as a slow start, we think that progress is being made and novel therapeutic tools will find their place in the armamentarium against MPM in the next decade.

SUMMARY

In the past decade, advances have been made that have improved the ability to treat MPM. There is evidence that these treatments are increasing the quality and quantity of life for patients with mesothelioma. Multimodality treatment programs that combine maximal surgical cytoreduction with novel forms of radiation therapy and more effective chemotherapy combinations may offer significant increases in survival for certain subgroups of patients with mesothelioma. Lung-sparing surgery may allow improvements in pulmonary function after surgery-based multimodality therapy, and potential longer overall survival than that seen with EPP. Experimental treatments such as immunotherapy and gene therapy provide hope for all patients with mesothelioma, and in the future may be combined with standard therapy in multimodality protocols.

REFERENCES

1. Antman KH, Pass HI, Li FP, et al. Benign and malignant mesothelioma, cancer. In: DeVita VT, Hellman S, Rosenberg S, editors. Principles and practice of oncology 4th edition, Philadelphia, PA: J.B. Lippincott Company; 1993. p. 1489–508.

2. Antman KH. Natural history and epidemiology of malignant mesothelioma. Chest 1993;103:373S.

3. Pisani RJ, Colby TV, Williams DE. Malignant mesothelioma of the pleura. Mayo Clin Proc 1988;63:1234.

4. Robinson BW, Lake RA. Advances in malignant mesothelioma. N Engl J Med 2005;353:1591–603.

5. Peto J, Hodgson JT, Matthews FE, et al. Continuing increase in mesothelioma mortality in Britain. Lancet 1995;345:535.

6. British Thoracic Society Standards of Care Committee. Statement on malignant mesothelioma in the United Kingdom. Thorax 2001;56:250.

7. Sterman DH, Kaiser LR, Albelda SM. Advances in the treatment of malignant pleural mesothelioma. Chest 1999;116:504–20.

8. Sterman DH, Albelda SM. Advances in the diagnosis, evaluation and management of malignant pleural mesothelioma. Respirology 2005;10:266–83.

9. Vogelzang NJ, Rusthoven JJ, Symanowski J, et al. Phase III study of pemetrexed in combination with cisplatin versus cisplatin alone in patients with malignant pleural mesothelioma. J Clin Oncol 2003;21:2636–44.

10. Haas AR, Sterman DH, Musani AI. Malignant pleural effusions: management options with consideration of coding, billing, and a decision approach. Chest 2007;132(3):1036–41.

11. Pien GW, Gant M, Washam C, et al. Use of an implantable pleural catheter for "trapped lung" syndrome in patients with malignant pleural effusion. Chest 2001;119:1641–6.

12. Lee YC, Fysh ET. Indwelling pleural catheter: changing the paradigm of malignant effusion management. J Thorac Oncol 2011;6(4):655–7.

13. Davies HE, Mishra EK, Kahan BC, et al. Effect of an indwelling pleural catheter vs chest tube and talc pleurodesis for relieving dyspnea in patients with malignant pleural effusion: the TIME2 randomized controlled trial. JAMA 2012;307(22):2383–9.

14. Waller DA, Morritt GN, Forty J. Video-assisted thoracoscopic pleurectomy in the management of malignant pleural effusion. Chest 1995;107:1454.

15. van Ruth S, Baas P, Zoetmulder FA. Surgical treatment of malignant pleural mesothelioma: a review. Chest 2003;123:551.

16. Rusch VW, Piantadosi S, Holmes EC. The role of extrapleural pneumonectomy in malignant pleural mesothelioma. A Lung Cancer Study Group trial. J Thorac Cardiovasc Surg 1991;102:1.

17. Sugarbaker DJ. Extrapleural pneumonectomy, chemotherapy and radiotherapy in the treatment of diffuse malignant pleural mesothelioma. J Thorac Cardiovasc Surg 1991;102:10.

18. Grondin SC, Sugarbaker DJ. Pleuropneumonectomy in the treatment of malignant pleural mesothelioma. Chest 1999;116:450S.

19. Sugarbaker DJ, Flores RM, Jaklitsch MT, et al. Resection margins, extrapleural nodal status, and cell type determine postoperative long-term survival in trimodality therapy of malignant pleural mesothelioma: results in 183 patients. J Thorac Cardiovasc Surg 1999;117:54.

20. Maggi G, Casadi C, Cianci R, et al. Trimodality management of malignant pleural mesothelioma. Eur J CardioThorac Surg 2001;19:346.

21. Sugarbaker DJ. Multimodality management of malignant pleural mesothelioma: introduction. Semin Thorac Cardiovasc Surg 2009;21(2):95–6.

22. Chang MY, Sugarbaker DJ. Innovative therapies: intraoperative intracavitary chemotherapy. Thorac Surg Clin 2004;14(4):549–56.

23. Tilleman TR, Richards WG, Zellos L, et al. Extrapleural pneumonectomy followed by intracavitary intraoperative hyperthermic cisplatin with pharmacologic cytoprotection for treatment of malignant pleural mesothelioma: a phase II prospective study. J Thorac Cardiovasc Surg 2009;138(2):405–11.

24. Bölükbas S, Manegold C, Eberlein M, et al. Survival after trimodality therapy for malignant pleural mesothelioma: radical pleurectomy, chemotherapy with cisplatin/pemetrexed and radiotherapy. Lung Cancer 2011;71:75–81.

25. Pass HI, Temeck BK, Kranda K, et al. Phase III randomized trial of surgery with or without intraoperative photodynamic therapy and postoperative immunochemotherapy for malignant pleural mesothelioma. Ann Surg Oncol 1997;4:628–33.

26. Friedberg JS, Mick R, Stevenson J, et al. A phase I study of Foscan-mediated photodynamic therapy and surgery in patients with mesothelioma. Ann Thorac Surg 2003;75:952–9.

27. Friedberg JS, Culligan MJ, Mick R, et al. Radical pleurectomy and intraoperative photodynamic therapy for malignant pleural mesothelioma. Ann Thorac Surg 2012;93(5):1658–65 [discussion: 1665–7].

28. Lang-Lazdunski L, Bille A, Belcher E, et al. Pleurectomy/decortication, hyperthermic pleural lavage with povidone-iodine followed by adjuvant chemotherapy in patients with malignant pleural mesothelioma. J Thorac Oncol 2011;6(10):1746–52.

29. Bölükbas S, Eberlein M, Schirren J. Prospective study on functional results after lung-sparing radical pleurectomy in the management of malignant pleural mesothelioma. J Thorac Oncol 2012;7(5):900–5.

30. de Graaf-Strukowska L, van der Zee J, van Putten W, et al. Factors influencing the outcome of radiotherapy in malignant mesothelioma of the pleura– a single institution experience with 189 patients. Int J Radiat Oncol Biol Phys 1999;43:511.

31. Boutin C, Rey F, Viallat JR. Prevention of malignant seeding after invasive diagnostic procedures in patients with pleural mesothelioma. Chest 1995;108:754.

32. Bydder S, Phillips M, Joseph DJ, et al. A randomised trial of single-dose radiotherapy to prevent procedure tract metastasis by malignant mesothelioma. Br J Cancer 2004;91:9.

33. Ahamad A, Stevens C, Smythe R, et al. Intensity-modulated radiation therapy: a novel approach to the management of malignant pleural mesothelioma. Int J Radiat Oncol Biol Phys 2003;55:768.

34. Ahamad A, Stevens C, Smythe R, et al. Promising early local control of malignant pleural mesothelioma following postoperative intensity modulated radiotherapy (IMTR) to the chest. Cancer J 2003;9:476.

35. Allen AM, Czerminska M, Jänne PA, et al. Fatal pneumonitis associated with intensity-modulated radiation therapy for mesothelioma. Int J Radiat Oncol Biol Phys 2006;65(3):640–5.

36. Janne PA. Chemotherapy for malignant pleural mesothelioma. Clin Lung Cancer 2003;5:98–106.

37. van Meerbeeck JP, Gaafar R, Manegold C, et al. Randomized phase III study of cisplatin with or without raltitrexed in patients with malignant pleural mesothelioma: an intergroup study of the European Organisation for Research and Treatment of Cancer Lung Cancer Group and the National Cancer Institute of Canada. J Clin Oncol 2005;23:6881–9.

38. Lee CW, Murray N, Anderson H, et al. Outcomes with first-line platinum-based combination chemotherapy for malignant pleural mesothelioma: a review of practice in British Columbia. Lung Cancer 2009; 64:308–13.

39. Ceresoli GL, Zucali PA, Favaretto AG, et al. Phase II study of pemetrexed plus carboplatin in malignant pleural mesothelioma. J Clin Oncol 2006;24: 1443–8.

40. Favaretto AG, Aversa SM, Paccagnella A, et al. Gemcitabine combined with carboplatin in patients with malignant pleural mesothelioma: a multicentric phase II study. Cancer 2003;97:2791–7.

41. Kindler HL, Karrison TG, Gandara DR, et al. Multicenter, double-blind, placebo-controlled, randomized phase II trial of gemcitabine/cisplatin plus bevacizumab or placebo inpatients with malignant mesothelioma. J Clin Oncol 2012;30(20):2509–15.

42. Zucali PA, Ceresoli GL, Garassino I, et al. Gemcitabine and vinorelbine in pemetrexed-pretreated patients with malignant pleural mesothelioma. Cancer 2008;112(7):1555–61.

43. Xanthopoulos A, Bauer TT, Blum TG, et al. Gemcitabine combined with oxaliplatin in pretreated patients with malignant pleural mesothelioma: an observational study. J Occup Med Toxicol 2008;3:34.

44. Stebbing J, Powles T, McPherson K, et al. The efficacy and safety of weekly vinorelbine in relapsed malignant pleural mesothelioma. Lung Cancer 2009;63:94–7.

45. Pasello G, Nicotra S, Marulli G, et al. Platinum-based doublet chemotherapy in pre-treated malignant pleural mesothelioma (MPM) patients: a mono-institutional experience. Lung Cancer 2011;73(3): 351–5.

46. Ceresoli GL, Zucali PA, De Vincenzo F, et al. Retreatment with pemetrexed-based chemotherapy in patients with malignant pleural mesothelioma. Lung Cancer 2011;72:73–7.

47. Zauderer MG, Krug LM. Novel therapies in phase II and III trials for malignant pleural mesothelioma. J Natl Compr Canc Netw 2012;10(1):42–7.

48. Mathy A, Baas P, Dalesio O, et al. Limited efficacy of imatinib mesylate in malignant mesothelioma: a phase II trial. Lung Cancer 2005;50:83.

49. Porta C, Mutti L, Tassi G. Negative results of an Italian Group for Mesothelioma (G.I.Me.) pilot study of single-agent imatinib mesylate in malignant pleural mesothelioma. Cancer Chemother Pharmacol 2007; 59:149.

50. Govindan R, Kratzke RA, Herndon JE 2nd, et al. Gefitinib in patients with malignant mesothelioma: a phase II study by the Cancer and Leukemia Group B. Clin Cancer Res 2005;11:2300.

51. Garland LL, Rankin C, Gandara DR, et al. Phase II study of erlotinib in patients with malignant pleural mesothelioma: a Southwest Oncology Group Study. J Clin Oncol 2007;25:2406.

52. Baas P, Boogerd W, Dalesio O, et al. Thalidomide in patients with malignant pleural mesothelioma. Lung Cancer 2005;48:291.

53. Dubey S, Janne PA, Krug L, et al. A phase II study of sorafenib in malignant mesothelioma: results of Cancer and Leukemia Group B 30307. J Thorac Oncol 2010;5:1655–61.

54. Ike O, Shimuzu V, Hitomi S, et al. Treatment of malignant pleural effusions with doxorubicin hydrochloride-containing ply (L-lactic acid) microspheres. Chest 1991;99:911.

55. Monneuse O, Beaujard AC, Guibert B, et al. Long-term results of intrathoracic chemohyperthermia (ITCH) for the treatment of pleural malignancies. Br J Cancer 2003;88:1839.

56. van Ruth S, Baas P, Haas RL, et al. Cytoreductive surgery combined with intraoperative hyperthermic intrathoracic chemotherapy for stage I malignant pleural mesothelioma. Ann Surg Oncol 2003;10: 176.

57. Bone G. Postoperative empyema and survival in lung cancer. Br Med J 1973;2(5859):178.

58. Minasian H, Lewis CT, Evans SJ. Influence of postoperative empyema on survival after pulmonary resection for bronchogenic carcinoma. Br Med J 1978;2(6148):1329–31.

59. Lawaetz O, Halkier E. The relationship between postoperative empyema and long-term survival after pneumonectomy. Results of surgical treatment of bronchogenic carcinoma. Scand J Thorac Cardiovasc Surg 1980;14(1):113–7.

60. Bakker W, Nijhuis-Heddes JM, van der Velde EA. Post-operative intrapleural BCG in lung cancer: a 5-year follow-up report. Cancer Immunol Immunother 1986;22(2):155–9.

61. Robinson BW, Manning LS, Bowman RV, et al. The scientific basis for the immunotherapy of human malignant mesothelioma. Eur Respir Rev 1993;3:195.

62. Astoul P, Picat-Joossen D, Viallat JR, et al. Intrapleural administration of interleukin-2 for the treatment of patients with malignant pleural mesothelioma: a phase II study. Cancer 1998;83:2099.

63. Boutin C, Nussbaum E, Monnet I, et al. Intrapleural treatment with recombinant gamma-interferon in early stage malignant mesothelioma. Cancer 1994; 74:2460.

64. Boutin C, Viallat JR, Van Zandwijk N, et al. Activity of intrapleural recombinant gamma-interferon in malignant mesothelioma. Cancer 1991;67:2033.

65. Goey SH, Eggermont AM, Punt CJ, et al. Intrapleural administration of interleukin 2 in pleural mesothelioma: a phase I-II study. Br J Cancer 1995;72:1283.

66. Nowak AK, Lake RA, Kindler HL, et al. New approaches for mesothelioma: biologics, vaccines, gene therapy, and other novel agents. Semin Oncol 2002;29:82.

67. Davidson JA, Musk AW, Wood BR, et al. Intralesional cytokine therapy in cancer: a pilot study of GM-CSF infusion in mesothelioma. J Immunother 1998;21(5): 389–98.

68. Vachani A, Moon E, Wakeam E, et al. Gene therapy for mesothelioma and lung cancer. Am J Respir Cell Mol Biol 2010;42(4):385–93.

69. Robinson BW, Mukherjee SA, Davidson A, et al. Cytokine gene therapy or infusion as treatment for solid human cancer. J Immunother 1998;21:211.

70. Hwang HC, Smythe WR, Elshami AA, et al. Gene therapy using adenovirus carrying the herpes simplex-thymidine kinase gene to treat in vivo models of human malignant mesothelioma and lung cancer. Am J Respir Cell Mol Biol 1995;13:7.

71. Smythe WR, Hwang HC, Amin KM, et al. Successful treatment of experimental human mesothelioma using adenovirus transfer of the herpes simplex-thymidine kinase gene. Ann Surg 1995;222:78.

72. Sterman D, Treat J, Litzky LA, et al. Adenovirus-mediated herpes simplex virus thymidine kinase/ganciclovir gene therapy in patients with localized malignancy: results of a phase I clinical trial in malignant mesothelioma. Hum Gene Ther 1998;9:1083.

73. Sterman DH, Molnar-Kimber K, Iyengar T, et al. A pilot study of systemic corticosteroid administration in conjunction with intrapleural adenoviral vector administration in patients with malignant pleural mesothelioma. Cancer Gene Ther 2000;7:1511.

74. Sterman DH, Recio A, Vachani A, et al. Long-term follow-up of patients with malignant pleural mesothelioma receiving high-dose adenovirus herpes simplex thymidine kinase/ganciclovir suicide gene therapy. Clin Cancer Res 2005;11(20):7444–53.

75. Schwarzenberger P, Lei DH, Freeman SM, et al. Antitumor activity with the HSV-tk-gene-modified cell line PA-1-STK in malignant mesothelioma. Am J Respir Cell Mol Biol 1998;19:333.

76. Schwarzenberger P, Byrne P, Gaumer R, et al. Treatment of mesothelioma with gene-modified PA1STK cells and ganciclovir: a phase I study. Cancer Gene Ther 2011;18(12):906–12.

77. Mukherjee S, Haenel T, Himbeck R, et al. Replication-restricted vaccinia as a cytokine gene therapy vector in cancer: persistent transgene expression despite antibody generation. Cancer Gene Ther 2000;7:663.

78. Odaka M, Sterman D, Wiewrodt R, et al. Eradication of intraperitoneal and distant tumor by adenovirus-mediated interferon-beta gene therapy due to induction of systemic immunity. Cancer Res 2001; 61:6201–12.

79. Vachani A, Sterman DH, Albelda SM. Cytokine gene therapy for malignant pleural mesothelioma. J Thorac Oncol 2007;2(4):265–7.

80. Sterman DH, Recio A, Carroll RG, et al. A phase I clinical trial of single-dose intrapleural IFN-beta gene transfer for malignant pleural mesothelioma and metastatic pleural effusions: high rate of anti-tumor immune responses. Clin Cancer Res 2007; 13:4456–66.

81. Sterman DH, Recio A, Haas AR, et al. A phase I trial of repeated intrapleural adenoviral-mediated interferon-beta gene transfer for mesothelioma and metastatic pleural effusions. Mol Ther 2010;18(4): 852–60.

82. Sterman DH, Haas AR, Moon E, et al. A trial of intrapleural adenoviral-mediated interferon-alpha2b gene transfer for malignant pleural mesothelioma. Am J Respir Crit Care Med 2011;184:1395–9.

83. Zhao Y, Moon E, Carpenito C, et al. Multiple injections of electroporated autologous T cells expressing a chimeric antigen receptor mediated regression of human disseminated tumor. Cancer Res 2010; 70(22):9053–61.

84. Dong M, Li X, Hong LJ, et al. Advanced malignant pleural or peritoneal effusion in patients treated with recombinant adenovirus p53 injection plus cisplatin. J Int Med Res 2008;36:1273–8.

Rare Pleural Tumors

Christopher T. Erb, MD, PhD[a], Kelsey M. Johnson, PA-C[b],
Anthony W. Kim, MD[c],*

KEYWORDS

- Primary pleural tumor • Pleural tumor • Solitary fibrous tumor of the pleura • Pleural effusion

KEY POINTS

- Primary pleural tumors are uncommon but are likely to be encountered in general clinical practice, prompting subspecialty referral.
- The diagnosis is established with proper imaging, tissue specimens, and histopathology and the adjunctive use of immunohistochemical staining and cytogenetics.

Primary pleural tumors are rare. By definition, they are benign or malignant lesions arising from either the parietal or visceral pleura. These tumors grow at variable rates and their prognosis is associated with the type and grade of tumor. Among primary pleural tumors, mesotheliomas predominate and these are discussed in detail elsewhere in this issue on pleural diseases in Clinics in Chest Medicine. The most common of the nonmesothelioma primary pleural tumors is solitary fibrous tumor of the pleura (SFTP). The other types comprise an exceedingly small proportion of the thoracic malignancies diagnosed each year in the United States and globally. As a consequence, the literature reviewing them consists primarily of case reports or small case series.

EPIDEMIOLOGY

Owing to the rarity of primary pleural tumors, many oncology texts and reviews do not include or discuss them in the context of thoracic cancers or cancer epidemiology.[1,2] It is estimated that the incidence of uncommon pleural tumors is approximately 2.8 cases per 100,000 hospitalizations in North America.[3] Malignant mesothelioma constitutes more than 90% of primary pleural tumors. Of the remaining 10%, approximately 5% are

classified as SFTPs and the other 5% are a variety of less common primary pleural tumors, such as lipomas, lymphomas, thymomas, melanomas, and sarcomas. Internationally, pleural tumors cause 0.3% to 3.5% of thoracic tumors.[3–6]

RISK FACTORS

Risk factors for nonmesothelioma primary pleural tumors are not well established. Primary pleural tumors do not seem to be as tightly linked to tobacco use as other more common lung cancers. A genetic syndrome has been implicated in some cases of rare pleural tumors, such as pleuropulmonary blastoma.[7] Gene mutations have been identified that may increase the risk for certain types of pleural tumors.[8,9] Other risks include radiation,[10] prior pleural interventions,[11] or chronic infection.[12] These are discussed in specific detail later in this article.

HISTOLOGIC FEATURES

The pleura is composed of a single layer of mesothelial cells that rest on a matrix of collagen, elastic fibers, blood vessels, and lymphatics.[13] Special foci of lymphoid tissue, called Kampmeier foci, may also be found along the pleural surface.[14] Tumors can arise from any of these cellular elements.

Disclosures: The authors have nothing to disclose.
a Section of Pulmonary, Critical Care, and Sleep Medicine, Department of Internal Medicine, Yale School of Medicine, 300 Cedar Street, TAC S-441, New Haven, CT 06520, USA; b Yale Thoracic Interventional Program, Smilow Cancer Hospital at Yale-New Haven Hospital, 15 York Street, LCI Suite 100, New Haven, CT 06510, USA; c Section of Thoracic Surgery, Yale School of Medicine, Thoracic Oncology Program, Smilow Cancer Hospital at Yale New Haven, 330 Cedar Street, BB 205, New Haven, CT 06520, USA
* Corresponding author.
E-mail address: anthony.kim@yale.edu

Clin Chest Med 34 (2013) 113–136
http://dx.doi.org/10.1016/j.ccm.2012.12.001

Primary pleural tumors are classified according to the World Health Organization (WHO) classification of lung tumors, last updated in 1999.[15] Pleural tumors are varied in histologic type, and fall under each of the broad categories of the WHO classification, including epithelial tumors, soft tissue tumors, mesothelial tumors, and miscellaneous tumors.[16] They can be divided into 4 major histologic categories based on their principal cellular appearance on light microscopy.[17] The 4 patterns are (1) spindle cell, (2) epithelioid, (3) biphasic (combined spindle and epithelioid pattern in one tumor), and (4) small blue cell. They can be further divided into 4 minor categories, including (1) papillary, (2) discohesive, (3) angiomatoid, and (4) lipomatous/clear cell pattern. Some will show mixed patterns, or cannot be fully characterized, but these classifications help to distinguish between benign and malignant primary pleural tumors versus metastatic disease.[17–19] Although the WHO classification does not yet incorporate immunohistochemical analysis and molecular studies, these are extremely useful and their importance is becoming recognized. Furthermore, additional cytogenetic testing for certain malignancies may also be useful in some cases.[20,21]

RADIOLOGIC FEATURES

There are few, if any, radiologic features that can absolutely distinguish benign from malignant primary pleural tumors or primary from metastatic tumors. Chest radiography is often followed by computed tomography (CT). Magnetic resonance imaging (MRI), positron emission tomography (PET or PET-CT), and ultrasonography (US) may also be used to help characterize the tumors and plan for further interventions, such as biopsy or surgical excision.

Chest Radiography

The chest radiograph is often the initial radiologic study obtained in the evaluation of pleural tumors, many of which are found incidentally. Some of the features that may help distinguish a benign from a malignant pleural tumor are circumferential or nodular thickening, a thickness greater than 1 cm, and involvement of the mediastinal pleura, which are all more commonly seen in malignant tumors. Effusions, when present, may be quite large and suggestive of malignancy.[22]

Chest CT

CT scan is the imaging technique of choice for characterizing the location, composition, and extent of pleural tumors.[10,23–25] Several features on CT scans may help distinguish tumors arising from the pleura from those arising from the lung parenchyma or elsewhere in the chest. The "incomplete border sign," an indistinct border toward the chest wall, but a sharp margin toward the lung, is helpful in distinguishing primary pleural from primary pulmonary tumors.[25,26] Tapered borders and an obtuse angle of interface with the chest wall or mediastinum, as opposed to an acute angle that is often seen with a peripheral mass arising from lung parenchyma, suggest primary pleural origin.[25]

CT scanning of the pleura is best done with intravenous contrast and should capture images from the thoracic inlet to the third lumbar vertebrae for complete visualization. Tissue phase imaging, rather than lung or bone windows, will provide the clearest images of the pleura.[27] CT scanning is better than chest radiography for detecting areas of necrosis, hemorrhage, calcification, and cystic changes, but may not be as good as MRI at distinguishing nodular structures, fluid-filled structures, or enhancement with contrast material.[28] CT scans have a reported sensitivity of 88% to 100% for detecting malignant pleural disease, but specificity is 40% to 45%.[29] Features on CT scans that are most helpful in distinguishing benign from malignant disease are the presence of a pleural rind, mediastinal pleural involvement, pleural nodularity, and invasion of adjacent structures.[30]

Ultrasonography

US may show well-defined, hypoechoic, solid, nodular lesions.[31–33] Tumors often have posterior acoustic enhancement and in some cases may be accompanied by atelectasis of the adjacent lung tissue.[34] By contrast, metastatic tumors or malignant mesothelioma may appear as more polypoid pleural nodules with sheetlike pleural thickening, often with an associated pleural effusion.[33] Malignant primary pleural tumors may exhibit irregular margins and deeper invasion of adjacent chest wall structures compared with their benign counterparts.[32]

US may not be able to distinguish primary pleural tumors from other tumors with pleural invasion, but may be useful in planning the diagnostic and therapeutic approach to pleural tumors, by localizing the tumor along the chest wall, and to guide transthoracic needle biopsy or thoracentesis.[33]

MRI

MRI is typically reserved for special scenarios unless a patient has an allergy to iodinated contrast dye.[27] However, MRI may help distinguish tissue planes and provide further information about invasion of adjacent structures[10] or tumor origin.[26] The soft tissue resolution and coronal and sagittal images offered by MRI may also reveal unique features of specific pleural tumors, such as peripheral rim enhancement, vascularity, or heterogeneity.[28] Gadolinium-based contrast material may highlight tumor-specific features. It is not first line because of the difficulty in performing and interpreting with respiratory and cardiac motion artifact.

PET and PET/CT

Generally, the PET scan has been used to detect metabolic activity and metastatic spread of cancer. Its use in the evaluation of primary pleural tumors has been less well studied because of these tumors' low incidence. Currently, PET may be best used to exclude another primary site of tumor as part of the evaluation of a suspected primary pleural tumor.[35,36] On fluorodeoxyglucose (FDG) PET-CT, pleural involvement may appear as localized, focal, or patchy FDG uptake, but this does not necessarily discern primary from metastatic disease, or local spread of primary lung carcinoma.[37–39] Some studies suggest that FDG PET-CT may be useful when distinguishing benign from malignant pleural tumors, with sensitivity, specificity, and negative predictive values between 88% and 96%.[36,40]

DISORDERS THAT MIMIC PRIMARY PLEURAL TUMORS ON CHEST IMAGING

Pleural-based tumors are often initially seen on routine chest radiographs or a CT scan obtained for some other purpose, and may be difficult to distinguish from other pleural-based processes. Because primary pleural tumors are so uncommon, these disorders are likely to be encountered in a general clinical practice,[41] and hopefully identified by an astute radiologist for referral to the thoracic specialist. **Table 1** lists several entities whose radiographic appearance may mimic primary pleural tumors, and **Fig. 1** shows characteristic images. These include pleural plaques, diffuse pleural thickening, rounded atelectasis, loculated pleural effusion, loculated hemothorax, extramedullary hematopoiesis, thoracic endometriosis with catamenial pneumothorax, thoracic splenosis, or metastatic malignancy. Non–pleural-based processes in proximity to the pleural surface, such as extrapleural hematoma, may also mimic rare pleural tumors.

When FDG PET-CT is the imaging modality used, there are several additional processes whose FDG avidity can mimic the appearance of malignant primary pleural tumors. These include

Table 1
Disorders that mimic primary pleural tumors on chest imaging

Entity	Distinguishing Features
Pleural plaques	Asbestos exposure; holly leaf shape on x-ray
Diffuse pleural thickening	Chronic inflammation; calcification; spans multiple ribs
Loculated pleural effusion	Biconvex opacity
Loculated hemothorax	May show a fluid-fluid level or increased attenuation
Loculate empyema	"Split pleura sign" with inflammation and hyper-enhancement
Extramedullary hematopoiesis	Rounded mass along a rib in patient with sickle cell disease or thalassemia
Rounded atelectasis	Focal, sharp-margined mass in patient with exposure to asbestos
Thoracic splenosis	Healed left rib fracture or history of trauma and an absent spleen
Metastatic disease	Usually multiple pleural-based nodules
Extrapleural hematoma	History of rib fracture; extrapleural fat displaced inward

inflammatory asbestos reactions, pleuritis from infections, sarcoidosis, and uremia, as well as changes associated with recent surgery or prior radiotherapy to the chest.[38]

DIAGNOSTIC APPROACH

The most important factor in the diagnosis of uncommon pleural tumors is to be aware of their possibility and have a high index of suspicion for their involvement. The imaging modalities, tissue sampling techniques, and histochemical analyses undertaken should be guided by the patient's clinical presentation and a thorough history and physical should be obtained, including demographics, risk factors, exposures, and associated symptoms and signs. When a suspicious pleural nodule or mass is identified, in addition to its detailed characterization, an exhaustive search for a primary lesion elsewhere should be pursued, as the vast majority of pleural tumors represent metastatic disease.[23,42] **Fig. 2** provides a diagnostic algorithm for the evaluation of a suspected primary pleural tumor.

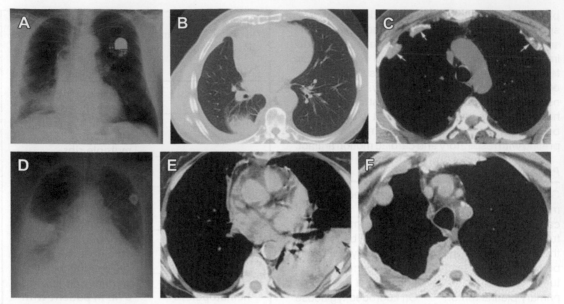

Fig. 1. Diseases resembling primary pleural tumors on imaging. (*A*, *B*) Rounded atelectasis, (*C*) pleural plaques (*arrows* indicate several anterior pleural plaques with calcification), (*D*) extramedullary hematopoiesis, (*E*) loculated haemothorax (*arrows* indicate areas of increased attenuation within the loculation), and (*F*) metastases from other primary tumors. ([*A*, *B*] *Courtesy of* Cindy R. Miller, MD, Associate Professor of Diagnostic Radiology, Yale School of Medicine, New Haven, CT; [*C*] *Adapted from* Nishimura SL, Broaddus VC. Asbestos-induced pleural disease. Clin Chest Med 1998;19(2):311–29; [*D*] *Courtesy of* Christopher T. Erb, MD, PhD, New Haven, CT; [*E*, *F*] *Adapted from* McLoud TC. CT and MR in pleural disease. Clin Chest Med 1998;19(2):261–76.)

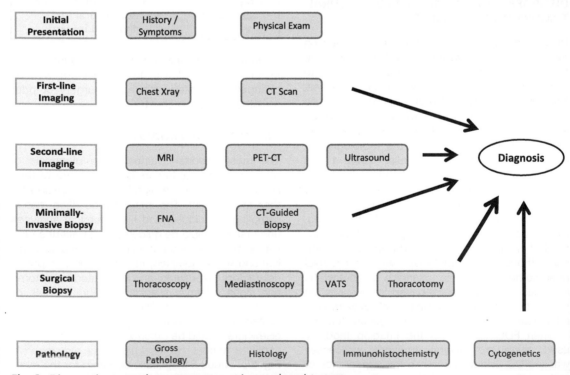

Fig. 2. Diagnostic approach to uncommon primary pleural tumors.

Securing a tissue diagnosis is of primary importance and can be achieved using a variety of modalities, including cytology, image-guided percutaneous biopsy, or surgical biopsy.[43] Two of the major challenges for the pathologist are differentiating malignant from reactive mesothelial cells and epithelioid mesothelioma from metastatic adenocarcinoma. Making this distinction often requires a tissue sample large enough to demonstrate the tumor's architecture and its pattern of attachment or invasion into surrounding structures.

If the tumor is associated with an effusion, draining the effusion for cytologic analysis of the pleural fluid may provide the simplest and most direct route to diagnosis.[44] However, cytology alone may be inadequate to distinguish neoplastic from reactive mesothelial cells, which may actually be more atypical and mitotically active.[43] Although it has not been studied specifically for rare primary pleural tumors, the diagnostic yield of pleural fluid sampling for suspected malignant effusions is reportedly between 49% and 60%. The diagnostic yield may be increased with serial pleural fluid sampling, and with the addition of percutaneous pleural biopsy,[45,46] or analysis of molecular markers.[47] When suspicion for malignancy is high, a negative cytologic result should be followed up with biopsy.[48,49]

Direct tissue sampling techniques include needle biopsy, core biopsy, image-guided biopsy, such as pleuroscopy, thoracoscopy or video-assisted thoracoscopic surgery (VATS), and thoracotomy.[43] The low sensitivity (50%) and negative predictive value (NPV) (33%) of needle biopsy make it less useful in many cases. However, CT or US-guided transthoracic biopsies are commonly used in the evaluation of primary pleural tumors, and their sensitivity is reportedly much higher (76%–87%).[50] Medical thoracoscopy (pleuroscopy) has a diagnostic yield of 97% for oxidative pleural effusions and a 100% NPV for excluding malignant effusions generally,[51] but has not been studied specifically for uncommon pleural tumors.

Surgical pleural biopsy via thoracoscopy or thoracotomy have been the gold standard for diagnosis of pleural malignancy with reported sensitivities of 94% to 98%,[52–54] and NPV of 93% to 100%.[55] VATS has been validated as an alternative to open thoracotomy for lobotomy in early-stage non–small-cell lung cancer,[56–58] but has not been studied specifically for primary pleural tumors because of their rarity. Nonetheless, it is commonly described as a diagnostic and therapeutic option in case reports of uncommon tumors of the pleura.

Newer alternatives to percutaneous sampling are evolving. The use of bronchoscope with or without end bronchial ultrasound (EBUS) has become more commonplace.[59]

Once a tissue sample is obtained, further analyses may include gross pathology, histology, immunohistochemistry, and in some cases, cytogenetics. More advanced testing will be guided by initial findings on gross pathology and histology, as some tumor types are easily identified under light microscopy or by primary histologic cell type alone.

TYPES OF PRIMARY PLEURAL TUMORS

Primary tumors that arise from the pleura can be benign or have varying degrees of malignant potential. Even benign tumors, however, will most often need to be resected and histopathological analysis undertaken to exclude their malignant counterparts (**Table 2**).

Table 2
Types of primary pleural tumors

Benign	Malignant
Solitary fibrous tumor (benign type)	Solitary fibrous tumor (malignant type)
Adenomatoid tumor	Primary pleural lymphoma
Calcifying fibrous tumor	Primary pleural thymoma
Lipoma	Primary pleural squamous cell carcinoma
Sclerosing hemangioma	Primary pleural melanoma
Schwannoma	Primary pleural sarcomas[a]
	Primitive neuroectodermal tumor of thoracopulmonary region (Askin tumor)
	Desmoid tumor
	Malignant peripheral nerve sheath tumor
	Desmoplastic small round cell tumor

[a] Includes vascular sarcoma, rhabdomyosarcoma, malignant fibrous histiocytoma, synovial sarcoma, osteosarcoma, liposarcoma, fibrosarcoma, chondrosarcoma, pleuropulmonary blastoma, and others.

SFTP

SFTPs represent about 5% of all pleural tumors, and are the most common primary pleural tumor after mesothelioma.[60] There are between 900 and 1760 cases of SFTP reported in the literature.[61,62] This large range is due to the variety of names used to describe them (localized fibrous tumor of the pleura, localized mesothelioma, localized fibrous mesothelioma, localized benign fibro, and submesothelial fibroma) and the controversy that existed around the taxonomy of these neoplasms for many decades, much of which centered around the cellular origin of these tumors.[63] Dedicated investigation and advancements in electron microscopy and immunohistochemical analysis has shown that SFTPs originate from the submesothelial mesenchymal layer of the pleura, which is thought to represent multipotential cells with limited ability to differentiate into mesothelial cells.[64]

SFTPs are usually benign, but in recent larger retrospective series, 7% to 43% of SFTPs have been reported to be malignant (**Table 3**).[61,65–70] These tumors can be found in patients from 5 to 87 years old, but are more commonly found in the fifth to sixth decade of life. In general, SFTPs are believed to affect men and women equally but some studies report a female preponderance. Unlike diffuse mesothelioma, exposures to asbestos or tobacco have not been found to be associated with SFTPs. Similarly, there are no familial links, although there is a case report of a mother and daughter who both developed an SFTP.[71]

Table 3
Studies of solitary fibrous tumor of the pleura providing data regarding benignity or malignancy and with more than 30 patients

Study	Total N	Benign (%)	Malignant (%)
Lahon[69]	157	90 (57)	67 (43)
Harrison-Phipps[68]	84	73 (87)	11 (13)
Magdeleinat[67]	60	38 (63)	22 (37)
Sung[61]	63	44 (70)	19 (30)
Cardillo[65]	110	95 (86)	15 (14)
Rosado-de-Christenson[26]	82	64 (78)	18 (22)
Guo[76]	39	35 (90)	4 (10)
Chu[77]	39	32 (82)	7 (18)
England[70]	223	141 (63)	82 (37)
Schirosi[84]	88	59 (67)	29 (33)
Total	945	671 (71)	274 (29)

Fewer than 40% of patients present with symptoms. When symptoms are present, the most common are cough (22%), dyspnea (22%), or chest pain (20%).[69] Serous pleural effusions have been reported.[65–67] SFTPs are also associated with 2 paraneoplastic syndromes: hypertrophic pulmonary osteoarthropathy (HPO or Pierre Marie-Bamberger syndrome) and hypoglycemia (Doege-Potter syndrome). It was initially believed that approximately 10% to 20% of patients with SFTPs presented with HPO; however, 2 recent large retrospective studies suggested a number closer to 2% to 3%.[62,65,69,70,72] HPO is thought to be caused by increased production of hyaluronic acid or hepatocyte growth factor resulting in periosteal changes, hypoxia, and secretion of cytokines. This can manifest as bilateral joint pain, swelling or stiffness, pain in the long bones, clubbing of the digits, hypertrophic skin changes, and, rarely, gynecomastia and galactorrhea. These syndromes disappear within hours to days following resection, with resolution of the clubbing and radiographic signs usually within 2 to 5 months.[66,73] Hypoglycemia is rare and thought to be caused by tumor secretion of an insulinlike growth factor type II that activates peripheral insulin receptors.[74] This abnormal secretion increases glucose uptake and prevents gluconeogenesis, causing refractory hypoglycemia.[75] Complete excision results in immediate resolution.[74]

SFTPs can grow to 39 cm and 62% are larger than 10 cm at presentation.[70] On chest radiography they may be well-circumscribed rounded nodules or occupy a substantial amount of the hemithorax. These tumors can arise anywhere in the chest, although some studies report that they more commonly arise in the inferior hemithorax.[26] They can also be found within the fissure, paravertebral, paramediastinal, or on the diaphragm, and they often have adhesions from the surface of the tumor to the opposing visceral or parietal pleura (**Table 4**).[70] If they originate on the diaphragm, they can be mistaken for an elevated hemidiaphragm. A pedunculated tumor can move with patient position or with serial imaging.[24,26] Most (74%) originate from the visceral pleura. It may be referred to as an "inverted fibroma" when it grows inward into the lung parenchyma (**Table 5**).[26,65,67–69,76,77]

On CT, SFTPs appear as a well-defined or lobulated solitary nodule or mass, and may manifest the "incomplete border sign," as shown in **Fig. 3**. Demonstration of a pedicle is helpful diagnostically, as well as for surgical planning, but is reported in only 25% of SFTPs.[78] Calcifications, chest wall involvement, or mass effect on adjacent structures have been observed, but are uncommon. Associated lymphadenopathy is typically not observed. They are heterogeneous with areas of increased

Table 4
Studies of solitary fibrous tumor of the pleura providing tumor location and with more than 30 patients

Study	Total N	Tumor Location Parietal (%)	Visceral (%)
Lahon[69]	157	40 (25)	117 (75)
Harrison-Phipps[68]	73[a]	15 (21)	58 (79)
Magdeleinat[67]	60	12 (20)	48 (80)
Cardillo[65]	110	15 (14)	95 (86)
Rosado-de-Christenson[26]	77	44 (57)	33 (43)
Guo[76]	39	15 (38)	24 (62)
Chu[77]	35[b]	8 (23)	27 (77)
Schirosi[84]	80[c]	15 (19)	65 (81)
Total	631	164 (26)	467 (74)

[a] Included 11 more patients; 4 of whom had tumors that were reported to arise from both pleura and 7 tumors were reported as intrapulmonary without visceral pleural involvement.
[b] Included 4 more patients who were reported as having solitary fibrous tumor of the pleura (SFTP) originate in the interstitial cells of the lung parenchyma.
[c] Included 8 more patients who were reported as having an intrapulmonary SFTP.

attenuation.[26] Tumors appearing homogeneous on CT scan are less common, usually smaller, and unlikely to be malignant.

MRI is rarely used. When performed, SFTPs typically appear as a low-intensity to intermediate-intensity mass on T1-weighted, T2-weighted, and proton density–weighted images, but signal intensity may be greater on T2-weighted compared with T1-weighted images.[26–28] The most helpful role of MRI is its ability to distinguish whether the SFTP is arising from the mediastinum, pericardium, or diaphragm.

Ultrasonography has been used to determine whether a lesion is above or below the diaphragm when other modalities are unable to do so.[79] The classic US appearance is a hypoechoic, well-circumscribed, oval, vascular mass situated between the lung and the pleura.[32]

Because these lesions tend to be highly vascularized, angiography may help to elucidate the origin of the tumor. Angiography has also been used preoperatively to embolize the tumor to mitigate potential bleeding at the time of resection.[80] There is little evidence to support the routine use of PET scans in the evaluation of SFTP. In one small series, PET scanning was associated with an 87.5% NPV for excluding malignant pleural disease.[65]

SFTPs are often described as a lobular mass with a smooth, glistening surface and significant vascularity on gross pathology. They also can have cystic, necrotic, or hemorrhagic areas interspersed.[26,70,81]

The best predictor of survival is complete resection.[69,70,81] Historically, the most common surgical approach was thoracotomy, but VATS is becoming more common, as expertise with this approach is improving (**Table 6**).[82] Specifically, VATS resection has been recommended for tumors that arise from the parietal pleura, are pedunculated, and are smaller than 2 cm, which was about 13% of cases in early series.[69] When using the VATS approach, caution should be taken

Table 5
Studies of solitary fibrous tumor of the pleura reporting tumor morphology and with more than 30 patients

Study	Total N	Morphology Pedunculated (%)	Sessile (%)	Inverted (%)
Lahon[69]	157	90 (57)	67 (43)	NR
Harrison-Phipps[68]	84	57 (68)	20 (24)	7 (8)[a]
Magdeleinat[67]	60	38 (63)	22 (37)	NR
Sung[61]	45	17 (38)	28 (62)	NR
Cardillo[65]	110	63 (57)	35 (32)	12 (11)
Rosado-de-Christenson[26]	65	38 (58)	27 (42)	NR
Guo[76]	39	16 (41)	23 (59)	NR
Chu[77]	35	29 (83)	6 (17)	NR
Schirosi[84]	88	55 (63)	25 (28)	8 (9)[a]
Total	683	403 (59)	253 (37)	27 (4)

Abbreviation: NR, not reported.
[a] Reported as "intrapulmonary."

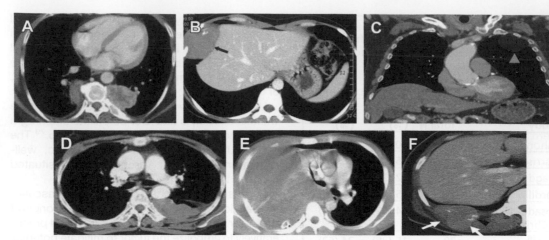

Fig. 3. Representative images of rare pleural tumors. (*A*) SFTP, (*B*) calcifying fibrous tumor of the pleura (*arrow* indicates the interface between the tumor and the diaphragm on the right), (*C*) CT scan showing coronal view of subpleural lipoma (arrowhead shows the homogenous hypodense pleural-based mass), (*D*) pleural thymoma, (*E*) primitive neuroectodermal tumor, and (*F*) pleural lymphoma (*arrows* indicate the soft tissue mass along the pleura; *arrowhead* indicates rib involvement with bony destruction). ([*A*] *From* Foran P, Colleran G, Madewell J, et al. Imaging of thoracic sarcomas of the chest wall, pleura, and lung. Semin in Ultrasound, CT, and MRI 2011;32(5):365–76; with permission; [*B*] *From* Jang KS, Oh YH, Han HX, et al. Calcifying fibrous pseudotumor of the pleura. Ann Thorac Surg 2004;78(6):e87–8; with permission; [*C*] *From* Karlo CA, Stolzmann P, Frauenfelder T, et al. Computed tomography imaging of subpleural lipoma in two men: two case reports. J Med Case Rep 2010;4:380; [*D*] *From* Kim HS, Lee HJ, Cho SY, et al. Myasthenia gravis in ectopic thymoma presenting as pleural masses. Lung Cancer 2007;57(1):115–7; with permission; [*E*] *Courtesy of* Cindy R. Miller, MD, Associate Professor of Diagnostic Radiology, Yale School of Medicine, New Haven, CT; and [*F*] *From* Bae YA, Lee KS. Cross-sectional evaluation of thoracic lymphoma. Thorac Surg Clin 2010;20(1):175–86.)

to avoid contact between the tumor and thoracoscopic sites because metastatic seeding and recurrence at port sites have been reported.[83] Sternotomy is often reserved for less common circumstances in which a thoracotomy or VATS would not provide adequate exposure.[61,65,67–69] Extended resections, including the chest wall, diaphragm, and multilevel hemivertebrectomies, have

Table 6
Studies of solitary fibrous tumor of the pleura reporting surgical approach and with more than 30 patients

Study	Total N	Surgical Approach			
		VATS	Thoracotomy	Sternotomy	Other
Harrison-Phipps[68]	84	12 (14)	68 (81)	3 (4)	1 (1)[a]
Magdeleinat[67]	60	6 (10)	53 (88)	1 (2)	0 (0)
Sung[61]	63	22 (35)	37 (59)	4 (6)	0 (0)
Cardillo[65]	110	69 (63)[b]	40 (36)	1 (1)	0 (0)
Guo[76]	39	9 (23)	30 (77)	0 (0)	0 (0)
Chu[77]	39	6 (15)	24 (62)	0 (0)	9 (23)[c]
Lahon[69]	157	20 (13)[d]	134 (85)	3 (2)	0 (0)
Total	552	144 (26)	386 (70)	12 (2)	10 (2)

Abbreviation: VATS, video-assisted thorascopic surgery.
 [a] Includes 1 patient with transabdominal approach for a hiatal mass that at the time of surgery was found to be a solitary fibrous tumor of the pleura.
 [b] Includes 16 patients whose surgery was converted to a thoracotomy.
 [c] Includes patients reported as undergoing "simple thoracoscopic surgery."
 [d] Includes 5 patients whose surgery was converted to a posterolateral thoracotomy.

been reported for en bloc resections used to achieve a negative margin.[69] Overall, operative morbidity and mortality vary from 0% to 12% and 0% to 4% respectively.[61,65,67–69]

Histologically, the most common pattern observed is a "patternless pattern." SFTPs also can exhibit a hemangiopericytomalike, storiform, herringbone, leiomyomalike, or neurofibromalike pattern (**Fig. 4**). Usually, SFTPs have a single histologic pattern (62%), but 2 (24%), or 3 (14%) or more patterns may also be observed.[70] SFTPs often have

ovoid or spindle-shaped cells with round to oval nuclei, small nucleoli, and faintly eosinophilic cytoplasm that is sometimes vacuolated.[70] Cellularity varies and collagen may form a fine lacelike network in cellular areas or appear in dense bundles and bands in hypocellular areas. Tumor cells can be found around branching capillaries and vessels, and occasionally entrapped bronchiolar, alveolar, and mesothelial epithelium may cause some confusion when trying to establish a diagnosis. Immunohistochemistry has proven helpful in differentiating

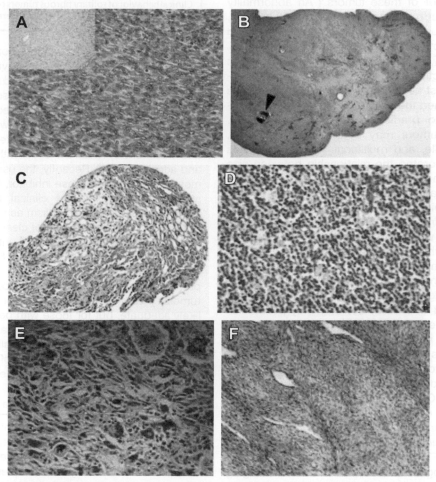

Fig. 4. (A) Histology of malignant solitary fibrous tumor of the pleura (SFTP) showing hypercellularity with a high mitotic index. In the inset, the characteristic hemangiopericytomalike pattern of the neoplasm is observed. (B) Calcifying fibrous tumor histopathology (hematoxylin-eosin [H&E] staining). Typically a nodular lesion with dense hyalinized collagen intermixed with calcified bodies (*arrowhead* indicates a calcified body, which stains dark with H&E). (C) Adenomatoid tumor histopathology (H&E staining). Loose collagen bundles surround ringlike vascular channels and epithelial inclusions. (D) Chest wall Askin (PNET) tumor (H&E staining). (E) Malignant fibrous histiocytoma (H&E staining). (F) Malignant peripheral nerve sheath tumor (H&E staining). (*From* [A] Cardillo G, Carbone L, Carleo F, et al. Solitary fibrous tumors of the pleura: an analysis of 110 patients treated in a single institution. Ann Thorac Surg 2009;88(5):1632–7; [B, C] English JC, Leslie KO. Pathology of the pleura. Clin Chest Med 2006;27(2):157–80; [D] Rais-Barhami S, Drabick JJ, De Marzo AM, et al, Xp11 translocation renal cell carcinoma: delayed but massive and lethal metastases of chemotherapy-associated secondary malignancy. Urology 2007;70(1):178.e3–6; and [E, F] Deniz K, Oban G, Okten T. Anti-CD10 [56C6] expression in soft tissue sarcomas. Pathol Res Pract 2012;208(5):281–5; with permission.)

SFTPs from other pleural tumors. They typically stain positive for vimentin, CD34, CD99, and Bcl-2 and negative for cytokeratin.[68,70,84]

Once the diagnosis is made, it is crucial to determine if the tumor is malignant and if its behavior is aggressive. The criteria for malignancy set forth by England and colleagues[70] includes (1) high mitotic activity (greater than 4 mitoses per high-power field), (2) high cellularity with crowding or overlapping of nuclei, (3) presence of necrosis, and (4) pleomorphism. Other factors, including cytogenetics, are being evaluated to better understand the biologic behavior of these tumors.[8] An abnormality on the long arm of chromosome 9, q22-33 region, may be important in the evolution, prognosis, and malignant potential of these tumors.[8]

Frequently the diagnosis of SFTP is not known before resection and whether an SFTP is malignant is almost never known a priori. Many studies have examined the clinical and radiographic characteristics to predict malignancy or benignity. Malignant tumors may be more symptomatic, larger, sessile, and multifocal.[69] Several studies have corroborated the relationship between size and malignancy.[61,65,68] Although a preoperative diagnosis may be helpful in some cases, the treatment of choice is the same for both benign and malignant tumors.

Patients with unresectable tumors usually succumb within 2 years to progressive disease.[85,86] Despite complete resection, up to two-thirds of malignant tumors exhibit local recurrence or metastasis.[70] Benign tumors recur in fewer than 5% of patients and when they do, they may present as a malignant lesion.[61,65,68,69,84] A median recurrence time of 34 months (malignant) and 83 months (benign) has been reported[68]; however, recurrences up to at least 6 years have occurred.[87] An increased risk of recurrence has been associated with CD34-negative tumors, tumors requiring an extensive surgical procedure, and sessile tumors.[69]

In a classic study, de Perrot and colleagues[88] classified SFTP on the basis of gross morphologic and pathologic features and created a staging system based the propensity for recurrence (**Box 1**). Malignant sessile tumors were most likely to recur (63%), followed by malignant pedunculated (14%), benign sessile (8%), and benign pedunculated (2%) tumors. The de Perrot staging system has correlated with several clinicopathologic parameters, including tumor necrosis, site of the tumor, pleomorphism, gross appearance, mitotic rate, multifocality, cellularity, and p53 expression.[84] Significant differences in 5-year survival between benign (96%) and malignant (68%) SFTPs have been observed.[69] Advanced

---

Box 1
Staging system of solitary fibrous tumors of the pleura

Stage 0: Benign pedunculated tumor

Stage I: Benign sessile or "inverted" tumor

Stage II: Malignant pedunculated tumor

Stage III: Malignant sessile or inverted tumor

Stage IV: Multiple synchronous metastatic tumors

Adapted from de Perrot M, Kurt AM, Robert JH, et al. Clinical behavior of solitary fibrous tumors of the pleura. Ann Thorac Surg 1999;67:1456–9; with permission.

---

stage and p53 overexpression correlate with a worse overall and disease-free survival.[84,88]

Because of the aforementioned recurrence rates, even after complete surgical resection, adjuvant therapies have been investigated. There are case reports of long-term survival with postsurgical radiation following incomplete resections and treatment of recurrent SFTP with ifosfamide and adriamycin.[89,90] Recently, the use of imatinib mesylate, a tyrosine kinase inhibitor, was associated with 21 months of clinical benefit and a decrease in tumor metabolism as measured by FDG-PET.[91] Despite the lack of clear evidence in favor of specific regimens, adjuvant therapy is now recommended for all malignant SFTPs.[72]

Long-term follow-up is recommended for all patients. For those with benign pedunculated tumors, yearly chest radiography or CT scan is likely adequate, but for those with benign sessile or malignant tumors, radiologic exams every 6 months for 2 years and then annually thereafter should be performed.[88] In the case of recurrence, repeat surgical resection is the treatment of choice.

Adenomatoid Tumor of the Pleura

Adenomatoid tumors are most commonly found arising from the genitourinary tract,[92] but may occur as primary pleural lesions as well. They typically present incidentally as small pleural nodules on chest imaging performed for another reason.[93,94] One case has been described in which the tumor was discovered during an intrathoracic operation for esophageal cancer and not visualized on preoperative imaging studies.[95] This tumor has not been associated with any known exposures and there is no reported sex difference. Surgical resection appears to be curative and they are not known to recur.

These benign tumors form nodular lesions up to 2 cm in diameter, are well circumscribed, and histologically are composed of tubules and dilated glandular structures, possibly with extensive vacuoles (see **Fig. 4**).[17,95] They have a relatively bland cytology, which makes them easy to distinguish from malignant tumors on pathologic examination.[95,96] Immunohistochemical stains confirm these tumors' mesothelial origin, and are typically positive for cytokeratin, vimentin, calretinin, and thrombomodulin, but negative for carcinoembryonic antigen (CEA), thyroid transcription factor-1 (TTF-1), epithelial membrane antigen (EMA), desmin, and CD34, among others.[95]

Calcifying Fibrous Tumor of the Pleura

Calcifying fibrous tumor of the pleura (CFT) has also been referred to as calcifying fibrous pseudotumor or disseminated calcifying tumor of the pleura in the 13 cases known to have been reported.[97–99] It is most common in young adults (mean age 35), but has been reported in patients in their fifth decade of life. No association has been found with smoking or asbestos exposure.[100] It may be more common among Japanese patients.[97] It is typically asymptomatic at presentation, but may be associated with chest pain.[101] Almost all cases have been identified incidentally after chest radiography or chest CT scanning has revealed a suspicious chest mass or pleural nodule (see **Fig. 3**), although it may present as multiple pleural nodules.[98]

Diagnosis is achieved by histopathology after surgical resection, and it must be distinguished from potentially malignant fibrous tumors, such as mesothelioma and metastatic sarcoma.[98] Surgical resection via VATS may be adequate to localize and remove the tumors,[97,99] but open thoracotomy may be necessary, especially when multiple lesions are seen or a malignant lesion is suspected.[98] Complete surgical removal is advised to prevent local recurrence or aggressive growth.[100]

CFTs are classified as soft tissue tumors under the WHO classification system.[15] Histologically, they appear as hyalinized dense collagenous tissue with lymphoplasmocytic infiltrates and calcifications and often contain psammoma bodies (see **Fig. 4**). They are almost universally positive for vimentin on immunohistochemical analysis, and exhibit variable positivity of other cellular markers, including factor XIIIa, smooth muscle actin (SMA), CD34, and osteopontin.[97] They are typically negative for S-100, desmin, and anaplastic lymphoma kinase.[99,102,103]

Pleural Lipoma

Lipomas are the most common benign tumors in adults, but primary pleural lipomas are exceedingly rare, with only 3 cases reported before 1970

and only 10 additional cases reported since that time, 5 of which were from one institution.[104] Most pleural lipomas are asymptomatic, but may present with chest pain, dyspnea, or even fever.[104] Digital clubbing is rare.[105] They are often discovered on routine chest imaging.[106]

On CT, they appear as round, solid tumors with a Hounsfield Unit density similar to subcutaneous adipose tissue (see **Fig. 3**).[24] They are homogeneous, lack calcifications, and do not enhance when contrast medium is injected.[107] They may resemble liposarcomas radiographically and sometimes on gross pathology, but they have no malignant potential.[104] There is one case reported of a fat-forming variant of SFTP with a similar radiographic appearance, but it was distinguished from a lipoma on CT by its heterogeneity and enhancement.[108] MRI is only rarely required to distinguish fascial planes and its lack of invasion into surrounding tissues.[24] PET-CT confirms its close association with the chest wall, but will show minimal uptake of FDG.[109]

Pleural lipomas are slow-growing tumors with no malignant potential, but surgical resection will sometimes be necessary if imaging cannot exclude malignant liposarcoma.[110] Furthermore, although historically managed conservatively, more recent recommendations favor early surgical resection even if the diagnosis is clearly established by chest CT because they can develop adhesions and become challenging to resect with interval growth, which can be quite large.[104] Resection via VATS or open thoracotomy have both been described.

The diagnosis usually may be accomplished via fine-needle aspiration (FNA), although complete surgical samples are often obtained.[110] Gross pathology reveals a smooth, yellowish mass that is encapsulated and may be lobulated.[106,111] Histologically, they consist of mature adipocytes without atypia.[112]

Sclerosing Hemangioma of the Pleura

Sclerosing hemangiomas are derived from incompletely differentiated respiratory epithelium. Consequently, updated nomenclature, such as pneumocytoma or sclerosing pneumocytoma, has been proposed, but the 1999 WHO classification did not vary from using the term sclerosing hemangioma.[15] More than 150 cases have been reported in the literature since the lesion was first described in 1956.[113,114]

Sclerosing hemangiomas are predominately asymptomatic, but hemoptysis, chronic cough, and chest pain have been reported.[114] There is a 5:1 female-to-male gender predilection, but no difference by race. The average age at diagnosis is 46 years. Metastases are quite uncommon at presentation, but even when present, do not affect survival.[115]

Sclerosing hemangiomas are almost always found incidentally on chest radiography, where they appear as small, solitary, noncavitating peripheral masses, typically smaller than 3 cm in diameter.[115] On CT scan they have smooth margins and may enhance with administration of contrast medium.[116]

Sclerosing hemangiomas are benign tumors treated with surgical excision without the need for additional treatment. No deaths have been associated with these tumors, although mean follow-up has been only 12 months (6–60 months) after resection in the largest series.[114]

The tumors have been found to be primarily of 2 cell types: surface cells and round cells. The surface cells resemble type II pneumocytes, whereas the round cells are small with scant chromatin and subtle nucleoli. Histologically, they are very heterogeneous, with areas of hemorrhage, inflammation, cystic spaces, calcifications, mast cells, hemosiderin, histiocytes, and accumulated surfactant.[115]

Immunohistochemical analysis is quite advanced in these tumors and typically confirms their origin as undifferentiated respiratory epithelium, defined by the presence of staining for TTF-1 and EMA and lack of reactivity to pancytokeratin, surfactant, and Clara cell markers.[114]

Primary Pleural Lymphoma

Primary pleural lymphomas make up only 2% to 7% of all lymphomas and may present as masses or as effusions, namely primary effusion lymphoma (PEL) or pyothorax-associated lymphoma (PAL). Pleural involvement by lymphoma typically represents spread of systemic disease.[96,117] Non-Hodgkins lymphoma is more likely than Hodgkins to be directly associated with the pleural surface. Presenting symptoms are nonspecific and most often include dyspnea and nonproductive cough. B-symptoms are less prominent than in systemic lymphoma.

PEL is thought to be caused by human herpes virus 8 or Epstein-Barr virus (EBV) and is found primarily in HIV-infected patients.[118] It presents as a pleural effusion, often without an identifiable tumor,[119] although it may be associated with plaquelike thickening of the pleura.[120] Mediastinal lymphadenopathy is rare.[121] PEL accounts for about 3% of AIDS-related lymphoma and fewer than 1% of lymphoma overall. Very rarely, mucosa-associated lymphoid tissue (MALT) and non–HIV-associated, non–pyothorax-associated primary pleural lymphoma have been reported.[121,122]

PAL is associated with chronic pyothorax in the setting of tubercular infection, often in combination with EBV infection.[12,96] It also has been described in patients with previous artificial pneumothorax used to treat tuberculosis.[123,124] Both PEL and PAL are predominantly diffuse large B-cell–type lymphomas.

CT scanning with administration of contrast material is recommended to help define tissues borders, subtle pleural-based changes, and to help guide tissue sampling (see **Fig. 3**). Primary pleural lymphoma commonly presents as a pleural-based mass that does not enhance with contrast, sometimes with destruction of adjacent bone.[120,125] Only about 10% are associated with pleural effusion at presentation.[117] MRI may occasionally be helpful to further characterize soft tissue masses and margins, including involvement of adjacent structures. PET or PET-CT may be superior to CT scan alone in detecting smaller tumors or areas of necrosis or fibrosis.[126] CT-guided biopsy is a common modality used to establish the diagnosis, but thoracoscopy may be necessary also.

Treatment involves surgical debulking if the tumor burden is high, followed by chemotherapy targeted at the specific tumor type identified by immunohistochemical analysis.[127] Chemotherapy typically includes standard regimens for B-cell lymphoma, including rituximab, cyclophosphamide, doxorubicin hydrochloride (hydroxydaunomycin), vincristine sulfate (Oncovin), Prednisone (R-CHOP).[119,120] Primary pleural lymphomas may be responsive to surgery and chemotherapy initially, but overall survival is low. Five-year survival of 50% after treatment has been reported.[119]

Tissue, histopathology, and immunostaining are all necessary to establish the diagnosis. The primary lymphoma type in both PEL and PAL is diffuse large B-cell, which typically stains positive for CD20, CD45, and CD79a and negative for CD5 and cyclin D1.[119,120] Follicular, marginal zone, and MALT have also been described.[119–121]

Primary Pleural Thymoma

Primary pleural thymomas tend to arise from the neck, mediastinum, or lung and generally make up fewer than 4% of all thymomas.[128–134] They usually present as an anterior mass, and may be quite large at the time of presentation. On chest radiography, a primary pleural thymoma may appear as diffuse nodular pleural thickening and initially can be confused with malignant mesothelioma (see **Fig. 3**).[131,135] Although myasthenia gravis is common in thymoma (30%–50% of cases), it is very rarely associated with primary pleural thymoma.[131] CT-guided core needle biopsy has been recommended over FNA given the higher diagnostic yield in some centers.

Surgical resection is recommended, but is not necessarily curative.[131,134] Complete surgical resection of both the primary tumor and the native thymic gland is recommended, followed by chemotherapy and radiation therapy as indicated by histologic grade and stage. Other treatment options may include cytoreductive surgery accompanied by hyperthermic intrathoracic chemotherapy, which has been shown to have 88% percent survival at the 22-month follow-up visit.[136] Indefinite regular surveillance for recurrence has been recommended.

Primary pleural thymomas can be distinguished from SFTP immunohistochemically by the lack of staining for CD34, vimentin, and BCL-2.[134] They also lack staining for CD5 and CD56, but may be positive for cytokeratin 19 and terminal deoxynucleotidyl transferase, suggesting their thymic cortical lymphocyte origins.[131]

Primitive Neuroectodermal Tumor

Askin tumor, or primitive neuroectodermal tumor (PNET), is a potentially aggressive soft tissue tumor of the pleura or chest wall that can be quite advanced at the time of diagnosis. It most frequently occurs in children and may be associated with the Ewing sarcoma family of tumors, based on its similar histology, immunohistochemistry, and cytogenetics.[137,138] First described in 1979 by Askin,[139] it was noted to have a female predominance and a very poor prognosis with a median survival of only 8 months. Presenting symptoms are nonspecific, but chest pain may be prominent, as the tumors are often large by the time of diagnosis. Other symptoms include cough, dyspnea, and weight loss.[140–142]

Chest radiographs typically show a pleural-based mass, sometimes with an associated effusion.[141,142] CT scanning may be useful for initial evaluation and detecting small pulmonary metastases, but Askin tumors are best evaluated with MRI. With this modality, they show sharp contrast enhancement, thus making it possible to distinguish tissue borders and tumor extension, even after chemotherapy.[143,144] T1, T2, and proton density imaging can be used for diagnosis and follow-up.[144] Larger tumors may appear heterogeneous on both CT and MRI, owing primarily to their tendency to form hemorrhage and necrosis (see **Fig. 3**).[142] Calcifications are rare.[137]

Management involves neoadjuvant chemotherapy, surgical excision, postoperative chemotherapy, and sometimes radiotherapy. Neoadjuvant chemotherapy increases the chances of obtaining a negative margin on surgical resection.[145] Radiotherapy is reserved for patients in whom negative surgical margins could not be obtained, typically because of large tumor burden with extension into the chest wall.[137] Survival has been reported to be 37% at 2 years and 14% at 6 years.[146]

Histologically, PNETs are composed of small round cells that contain neurosecretory granules and Homer-Wright rosettes, and stain positive for neuron-specific enolase, MIC2, CD99, and vimentin (see **Fig. 4**). Its histology is not unique and therefore requires immunohistochemical analysis and electron microscopy to distinguish definitively.[147] Cytogenetic testing is helpful if an Askin tumor is suspected, as a chromosomal translocation has been identified: t(11;22)(q24:q12).[9]

Squamous Cell Carcinoma of the Pleura

Approximately 9 cases of primary squamous cell carcinoma (SCC) of the pleura have been reported.[11] Early associations were found between chronically draining empyema[148] and extrapleural pneumolysis for pulmonary tuberculosis in which the adjacent metaplastic mesothelial cells of the pleura transformed to SCC.[149] More recently, primary pleural SCC has been reported in association with a persistent bronchopleural fistula after an Eloesser procedure.[11] Prior pneumonectomy, primarily as treatment for tuberculosis, also has been reported to be a unique association,11 with delays in development of SCC lagging by as many as 20 years from the original procedure. As such, these primary pleural tumors are thought to arise in areas of chronic inflammation.[150]

Chest pain is the most common presenting complaint. Pleural thickening may be the only radiographic sign in the area of chronic changes.[11] Pleural biopsy reveals keratinized, well-differentiated, stratified squamous epidermal cells that are typical of SCC. As with squamous cell carcinomas arising elsewhere, prognosis is poor and complete excision followed by radiation therapy is typically offered.

Primary Pleural Malignant Melanoma

Melanoma makes up approximately 1% of all malignant tumors, but primary pleural involvement is an exceptionally rare presentation, with fewer than 10 cases reported. First reported in 1978, its occurrence has been postulated to be related to early fetal migration of melanocytes concurrently with primordial tubular respiratory tract cells to the pleural lining.[151–154] They may be associated with congenital abnormalities, such as congenital hairy nevus syndrome.[152] Symptoms may include dyspnea, productive cough, and anorexia with weight loss.[152,155] When a pleural melanoma is identified, an extensive search for an alternative primary site is critical, including a surgical and dermatologic history, physical examination, and diagnostic imaging.[153,154]

Chest radiography may show nodular soft tissue thickening in any area of the pleural lining, a pleural effusion, and occasionally complete opacification of the hemithorax associated with mediastinal shift.[152] CT may detect an often sizable pleural-based mass associated with an ipsilateral pleural effusion.[155] PET scanning may help exclude metastatic disease.[156]

Once a diagnosis is established, chemotherapy targeted at melanoma should be initiated. Response and recurrence can be followed with serial CT scans. As with malignant melanomas at other primary sites, the prognosis is poor, with the survival reported to be on the order of months.[155,156]

Pleural fluid cytology may be enough to diagnosis the lesion, especially if the typical findings of degenerated mesothelial cells with a large nucleus, coarse chromatin, and scant cytoplasm containing coarse blackish-brown pigment are present.[152,155] On histopathology, there is abundant intracellular and extracellular melanin deposition, and on immunohistochemical staining, positivity for S-100 and HMB-45 is seen, confirming the diagnosis of melanoma.[152,155,157]

Primary Pleural Sarcomas

Sarcomas may arise from any element of pleural tissue, and many are mixed forms with more than one cell type involved.[158] Embryologically, they arise from pluripotent stem cells that become neoplastic and diverge into epithelial or sarcomatous components.[7] As a class, sarcomas have also been referred to as spindle cell tumors because of their histologic patterns.[159] They are quite rare and are often initially mistaken for malignant mesothelioma, metastatic carcinoma, or other nonmalignant processes.[10,42,160–167]

Sarcomas of almost all histologic varieties have been reported as cases or case series, often with very few total numbers.[168–174] As a group, they have similar clinical presentation, radiologic features, and gross pathologic appearance, and can be diagnosed definitively only with immunohistochemical analysis or cytogenetics.[10] Similar to sarcomas elsewhere, the prognosis is quite poor.[161,165]

The initial clinical presentation of patients with a primary pleural sarcoma is nonspecific, with cough, dyspnea, and chest pain being the most common symptoms reported.[28,162,172,174–176] Fevers and chills may be present.[171,173,177]

Angiosarcomas may present with a haemothorax.[160,161,166] Risk factors for certain pleural sarcomas include history of chest wall irradiation, chronic tuberculous pyothorax,[165] asbestos exposure,[173,178] and smoking.[179]

Chest radiography typically reveals pleural thickening and there may be an extensive effusion present.[22,165,166,176,180] US may also reveal an effusion or echogenic heterogeneous soft tissue mass with necrosis.[177] CT imaging may be helpful in narrowing the differential diagnosis on the basis of location, vascularity, calcification, or heterogeneity (see **Fig. 3**).[28] Tumors often appear as solid, high-density masses, but they may have areas of necrosis, hemorrhage, increased vascularity, or calcification.[22] PET-CT may suggest the malignant potential, biologic activity, and primary location of the lesion, but tissue sampling is essential. FNA is typically nondiagnostic, and although CT-guided transthoracic biopsy may be diagnostic in rare cases,[181] surgical biopsy and complete tumor excision are recommended.[22,173,182] Chemotherapy and radiation therapy are often recommended[172,174,183] and close follow-up is warranted, as recurrence is common.

As suggested previously, histologic subtypes include leiomyosarcoma, malignant fibrous histiosarcoma (MFH), fibrosarcoma, synovial sarcoma, angiosarcoma, rhabdomyosarcoma, chondrosarcoma, osteosarcoma, or an undifferentiated subtype.[159,163,184] Occasionally, histologic analysis alone will be sufficient to arrive at a definitive diagnosis, as in the case of liposarcoma, but in most cases further analysis with immunohistochemical or cytogenetic analysis will be required. Immunohistochemical staining for cytokeratin, vimentin, calretinin, CD34, CD99, EMA, Bcl-2, S-100, and desmin can be performed. The classic immunohistochemical pattern for sarcomas is positive staining for vimentin and negative staining for cytokeratins.[161] An individual tumor's profile may include positive staining for additional markers, and these variations may help to distinguish the subtype of sarcomas or exclude another type of tumor.[185] The rest of this section reviews immunochemical stains, although these are summarized in (**Table 7**). Carcinomas will typically be positive for pankeratin markers, CEA, and thrombomodulin, and negative for calretinin.[175] By contrast, typical mesothelial cell markers include cytokeratin 5/6, calretinin, and WT1, whereas typical epithelial/adenocarcinoma markers include Ber-EP4, CEA, and TTF-1. Cytokeratin is also positive in the mesothelioma variants and in synovial sarcoma.[17] CD31 may be the most sensitive and specific for angiosarcoma.[176,185] SFTPs are classically positive for CD34, CD99, and Bcl-2, in addition to

Table 7
Immunohistochemical analysis of primary pleural sarcomas and comparison to solitary fibrous tumor of the pleura and carcinomas

Tumor Type	Vimentin	Cytokeratin	Desmin	Actin	EMA	S-100	C99	Factor 8	Calretinin	SMA	Bcl-2	CD31	CD34	CEA	TTF-1
SFTP	+	-	-	-	-	-	+	-	-	-	+	-	+	-	-
Carcinoma	-	+	-	-	-	-	-	-	-	-	-	-	-	+	+
Primary smooth muscle tumor	+	-	+	+	-	-	-	-	-	+	-	-	+/-	-	-
Vascular sarcoma	+	-	-	-	-	-	-	+	-	-	-	+	-	-	-
Rhabdomyosarcoma	+	-	+	-	-	-	-	-	-	-	-	-	-	-	-
Malignant fibrous histiocytoma	+	-	-	-	-	-	-	-	+	-	-	-	-	-	-
Synovial sarcoma	+	+/-	-	-	+	-	+	-	-	-	+	-	-	+	-
Liposarcoma	+	-	-	-	-	-	-	-	-	-	-	-	-	-	-
Fibrosarcoma	+	-	-	-	-	+	-	-	-	-	+	-	-	-	-
Epithelioid hemangioendothelioma	+	-	-	-	-	-	-	+	-	-	-	+	+	-	-
Chondrosarcoma	+	-	-	+	-	+	+	-	+	-	-	-	-	-	-

(+) indicates the marker is typically positive in the tumor type indicated; (−) indicates the marker is typically negative in the tumor type indicated; (-) indicates the marker is not routinely tested for in the work up or a particular tumor type, but would presumably be negative if it were to be tested for.

Abbreviations: CEA, carcinoembryonic antigen; EMA, epithelial membrane antigen; SFTP, solitary fibrous tumor of the pleura; SMA, smooth muscle actin; TTF-1, thyroid transcription factor-1.

vimentin.[70–77,84] EMA is present only in synovial sarcoma and S-100 differentiates schwannoma from the others in the group.[17,186] Absence of typical cytologic markers of carcinoma, such as CEA and TTF-1, may be helpful in excluding metastasis of another primary tumor.[95]

Primary smooth muscle tumors of the pleura, including leiomyoma and leiomyosarcoma, will show bland spindle cell with features of muscular differentiation and will stain positive for vimentin, alpha-SMA, desmin, HHF-35, smooth muscle myosin-heavy chain, and occasionally weak focal positivity for keratin and CD34.[187–190] Smooth muscle tumors are negative for S-100, Bcl-2, CD99, and most of the cytokeratin panel.[189] Soft tissue leiomyosarcomas commonly have chromosomal losses at 10q and 13q.[187] Myopericytomas will be positive for vimentin, SMA, muscle-specific actin, and Bcl-2; negative for desmin, h-caldesmon, cytokeratin, and CD34; and will have a characteristic perivascular arrangement of spindle cells.[191]

Vascular tumors, such as angiosarcomas, will show positivity for vimentin and be negative or only focally positive for cytokeratin.[165,176] When this pattern is observed, additional vascular markers, such as CD34, CD31, and factor VIII, can be used to confirm the diagnosis. Of these, CD31 is the most sensitive and specific.[185] CD31 is almost universally positive in angiosarcomas and if present in a tumor of epithelioid histology, is essentially diagnostic of angiosarcoma.[165,166]

Rhabdomyosarcomas will stain for myoglobin (myoD1), desmin, vimentin, and creatinine phosphokinase-MM and may be differentiated radiographically from Ewing sarcoma in that they rarely involve the ribs.[177,192,193]

Malignant fibrous histiocytoma may be positive for vimentin, CD68, lysozyme, and calretinin and negative for cytokeratin, EMA, SMA, and desmin.[194,195]

Synovial sarcomas will be positive for vimentin, Bcl-2, and CD99, helping distinguish them from malignant mesothelioma.[196,197] They may also show focal positivity within sarcomatous elements for keratin and EMA, and express mucin and the carcinoma markers Ber-EP4, CEA, and AUA1.[20,196–198]

Osteosarcomas may not require immunohistochemical staining, as they may completely replace pleural tissue with bony material that is readily identifiable on light microscopy by islands of malignant osteoid without epithelial or mesothelial elements.[199,200]

Liposarcomas will show the typical sarcoma pattern of positivity to vimentin and negativity to cytokeratin. They are also commonly negative for EMA, desmin, and actin.[184]

Fibrosarcomas of the pleura will stain positive for vimentin, S-100, and possibly Bcl-2, but negative for all other markers.[201] They are also associated with a pathognomonic gene translocation (t[7;16][q33;p11]), which results in a fusion gene transcript known as FUS-CREB3L2.[201–203] Desmoid tumors are considered a variant of low-grade fibrosarcoma and will typically stain positive for vimentin and SMA, may stain positive for desmin and muscle-specific actin,[186] but stain negative for CD34 and S-100.[204]

Epithelioid hemangioendothelioma is a vascular tumor with poor prognosis that can be distinguished by positivity for vimentin, CD31, CD34, and Factor VIII, and negativity for cytokeratin, calretinin, CEA, TTF-1, WT-1, and S-100.[205–207] On electron microscopy, Weibel-Palade bodies are apparent.[208]

Chondrosarcomas will typically stain positive for S-100, CD99, vimentin, actin, lysozyme, and sometimes p53, but negative for CD34, desmin, EMA, calretinin, CEA, factor VIII, and cytokeratins. They will also have a high content of cartilaginous material such as chondroitin 4-sulfate and 6-sulfate.[173,178,181]

Possible primary pleural sarcomas also need to be distinguished from heterologous mesothelioma, which is characterized by inclusion of osteosarcomatous, chondrosarcomatous, or rhabdomyoblastic histologic elements, but by immunohistochemical analysis that is typical of mesothelioma.[209]

Additional cytogenetic testing for certain malignancies (ie, chromosomal translocation t[X;18] in synovial sarcoma) may also be useful in some cases.[20,21,210] DICER1 and p53 mutations have been identified in patients with pleuropulmonary blastoma.[7,211,212]

Other Rare Pleural Tumors

A few other primary pleural tumors have been rarely described in the literature. Desmoplastic small round cell tumor (DSRCT) is classically an intra-abdominal tumor, but has been described several times arising from the pleura. It presents nonspecifically, usually in younger adults. It is composed of small poorly differentiated malignant cells associated with desmoplastic stromal cells that stain positive for epithelial (cytokeratins), mesenchymal (vimentin, desmin), and neuroendocrine (chromogranin and neuron-specific enolase) markers.[213–215] It is the positive staining for desmin that distinguishes it from other tumors with a biphasic pattern.[17] Cytologic analysis of pleural fluid is often enough to make the diagnosis if the proper immunohistochemical staining is performed.[215] The EWS-WT1 translocation (t[11;22][q13;q12]) is also characteristic of DSRCT and has been shown to occur in the pleura-based tumors.[213] Multimodal treatment, including chemotherapy, radiotherapy, and surgical resection, has been advocated.[216] It is a very aggressive tumor and life expectancy is on the order of months to a few years.[214,216]

Benign schwannomas and their counterparts, the malignant peripheral nerve sheath tumors, have also been reported to arise directly from the pleura. Typically arising from an intercostal nerve in the posterior-superior mediastinum, they extend along the parietal pleura and may grow to be quite large.[217] They may be associated with a bloody pleural effusion or hemothorax.[218] One case has been reported in association with type II neurofibromatosis[219] and another after exposure to radiation therapy for Hodgkin disease.[220] Immunohistochemical staining can help confirm the diagnosis, as this spindle cell tumor typically stains positive for S-100 and vimentin and negative for CD34, SMA, and cytokeratin.

SUMMARY

Primary pleural tumors are uncommon but are likely to be encountered in general clinical practice, prompting subspecialty referral. The diagnosis is established with proper imaging, tissue specimens, and histopathology, and the adjunctive use of immunohistochemical staining and cytogenetics. In this article, we have described the radiographic and pathologic features of the less common primary pleural tumors and proposed a diagnostic approach to their evaluation.

REFERENCES

1. Dela Cruz CS. Lung cancer: epidemiology, etiology, and prevention. Clin Chest Med 2011;32: 605–44.
2. DeVita VT, Lawrence TS, Rosenberg SA, et al. In: DeVita, Hellman, Rosenberg, editors. Cancer: principles & practice of oncology. 9th edition. Lippincott Williams & Wilkins (LWW); 2011.
3. Furrer M, Inderbitzi R. Case report: endoscopic resection of a 5 cm intrathoracic lipoma. Pneumologie 1992;46:334–5 [in German].
4. Sekine I, Kodama T, Yokose T, et al. Rare pulmonary tumors—a review of 32 cases. Oncology 1998;55(5):431–4.
5. Grigor'eva SP, Revzis MG. Rare malignant tumors of the lungs (44 cases). Vopr Onkol 1979;25(2). 24–23. [in Russian].
6. Nitsche K, Günther B, Katenkamp D, et al. Thoracic neoplasms at the Jena reference center for soft tissue tumors. J Cancer Res Clin Oncol 2012; 138(3):415–24.
7. Travis WD. Sarcomatoid neoplasms of the lung and pleura. Arch Pathol Lab Med 2010;134: 1645–58.
8. Torres-Olivera FJ, Vargas MT, Torres-Gomez FJ, et al. Cytogenetic, fluorescence in situ hybridization, and immunohistochemistry studies in a malignant pleural solitary fibrous tumor. Cancer Genet Cytogenet 2009;189:122–6.
9. Delattre O, Zucman J, Melot T, et al. The Ewing family of tumors—a subgroup of small-round-cell tumors defined by specific chimeric transcripts. N Engl J Med 1994;331(5):294–9.
10. Gladish GW, Sabloff BM, Munden RF, et al. Primary thoracic sarcomas. Radiographics 2002;22(3): 621–37.
11. Franke M, Chung H, Johnson FE. Squamous cell carcinoma arising from the pleura after pneumonectomy for squamous cell carcinoma of the lung. Am J Surg 2010;199:e34–5.
12. Molinie V, Pouchot J, Navratil E, et al. Primary Epstein-Barr virus-related non-Hodgkin's lymphoma of the pleural cavity following long-standing tuberculous empyema. Arch Pathol Lab Med 1996;120(3):288–91.
13. Finley DJ, Rusch VW. Anatomy of the pleura. Thorac Surg Clin 2011;21(2):157–63.
14. Wang NS. Anatomy of the pleura. Clin Chest Med 1998;19(2):229–40.
15. Travis WD, Colby TV, Corrin B, et al. In Collaboration with Sobin LH and Pathologists from 14 Countries. World Health Organization International Histological Classification of Tumours. Histological Typing of Lung and Pleural Tumours. 3rd edition. Springer-Verlag; 1999.
16. Brambilla E, Travis WD, Colby RV, et al. The new World Health Organization classification of lung tumours. Eur Respir J 2001;18:1059–68.
17. Granville L, Laga AC, Allen TC, et al. Review and update of uncommon primary pleural tumors: a practical approach to diagnosis. Arch Pathol Lab Med 2005;129:1428–43.
18. Ordonez N. The diagnostic utility of immunohistochemistry in distinguishing between mesothelioma and renal cell carcinoma: a comparative study. Hum Pathol 2004;35;697–710.
19. Flieder DB, Moran CA, Travis WD, et al. Pleuropulmonary endometriosis and pulmonary ectopic deciduosis: a clinicopathologic and immunohistochemical study of 10 cases with emphasis on diagnostic pitfalls. Hum Pathol 1998;29:1495–503.
20. Begueret H, Galateau-Salle F, Guillou L, et al. Primary intrathoracic synovial sarcoma: a clinicopathologic study of 40 t(X;18)-positive cases from the French Sarcoma Group and the Mesopath Group. Am J Surg Pathol 2005;29(3):339–46.

21. Colwell AS, D'Cunha J, Vargas SO, et al. Synovial sarcoma of the pleura: a clinical and pathologic study of three cases. J Thorac Cardiovasc Surg 2002;124:828–32.

22. Baisi A, Raveglia F, De Simone M, et al. Primary multifocal angiosarcoma of the pleura. Interact Cardiovasc Thorac Surg 2011;12:1069–70.

23. Salahudeen HM, Hoey ET, Robertson RJ, et al. CT appearances of pleural tumors. Clin Radiol 2009; 64(9):918–30.

24. McLoud T. CT and MRI in pleural disease. Clin Chest Med 1998;19(2):261–76.

25. Dynes MC, White EM, Fry WA, et al. Imaging manifestations of pleural tumors. Radiographics 1992; 12(6):1191–201.

26. Rosado-de-Christenson ML, Abbott GF, McAdams HP, et al. From the Archives of the AFIP: localized fibrous tumors of the pleura. Radiographics 2003;23:759–83.

27. Helm EJ, Matin TN, Gleeson FV. Imaging of the pleura. J Magn Reson Imaging 2010;32:1275–86.

28. Foran P, Colleran G, Madewell J, et al. Imaging of thoracic sarcomas of the chest wall, pleura, and lung. Semin Ultrasound CT MR 2011;32:365–76.

29. Leung AN, Muller NL, Miller RR. CT in differential diagnosis of diffuse pleural disease. Am J Roentgenol 1990;154(3):487–92.

30. Metintas M, Ucgun I, Elbek O, et al. Computed tomography features in malignant pleural mesothelioma and other commonly seen pleural diseases. Eur J Radiol 2002;41(1):1–9.

31. Hew M, Heinze S. Chest ultrasound in practice: a review of utility in the clinical setting. Intern Med J 2012;42(8):856–65.

32. Chira R, Chira A, Mircea PA. Thoracic wall ultrasonography—normal and pathological findings. Pictorial essay. Med Ultrason 2011;13(3):228–33.

33. Tsai TH, Yang PC. Ultrasound in the diagnosis and management of pleural disease. Curr Opin Pulm Med 2003;9:282–90.

34. Rumende CM. The role of ultrasonography in the management of lung and pleural diseases. Acta Med Indones 2012;44(2):175–83.

35. Duranti L, Leo F, Pastorino U. PET scan contribution in chest tumor management: a systematic review for thoracic surgeons. Tumori 2012;98(2): 175–84.

36. Duysinx B, Nguyen D, Louis R, et al. Evaluation of pleural disease with 18-fluorodeoxyglucose positron emission tomography imaging. Chest 2004; 125(2):489–93.

37. Hara M, Oshima H, Suzuki H, et al. The frontiers of diagnostic radiology –PET/CT, 3DCT. Nihon Geka Gakkai Zasshi 2005;106(11):677–84 [in Japanese].

38. Makis W, Ciarallo A, Hickeson M, et al. Spectrum of malignant pleural and pericardial disease on FDG PET/CT. Am J Radiol 2012;198:678–85.

39. Mavi A, Lakhani P, Zhuang H, et al. Fluorodeoxyglucose-PET in characterizing solitary pulmonary nodules, assessing pleural diseases, and the initial staging, restaging, therapy planning, and monitoring response of lung cancer. Radiol Clin North Am 2005;43(1):1–21.

40. Alavi A, Gupta N, Alberini JL, et al. Positron emission tomography imaging in nonmalignant thoracic disorders. Semin Nucl Med 2001;32(4):293–321.

41. Walker CM, Takasugi JE, Chung JH, et al. Tumorlike conditions of the pleura. Radiographics 2012; 32(4):971–85.

42. Ruhland B, Dittmer C, Thill M, et al. Metastasized hemangiopericytoma of the breast: a rare case. Arch Gynecol Obstet 2009;280(3):491–4.

43. Andrews TD, Wallace WA. Diagnosis and staging of lung and pleural malignancy—an overview of tissue sampling techniques and the implications for pathological assessment. Clin Oncol 2009;21:451–63.

44. Cakir E, Demirag F, Aydin M, et al. A review of uncommon cytopathologic diagnoses of pleural effusions from a chest disease center in Turkey. Cytojournal 2011;8:13.

45. Ong KC, Indumathi V, Poh WT, et al. The diagnostic yield of pleural fluid cytology in malignant pleural effusions. Singapore Med J 2000;41(1):19–23.

46. Fenton KN, Richardson JD. Diagnosis and management of malignant pleural effusions. Am J Surg 1995;170:69–74.

47. Brock MV, Hooker CM, Yung R, et al. Can we improve the cytologic examination of malignant pleural effusions using molecular analysis? Ann Thorac Surg 2005;80:1241–7.

48. Renshaw AA, Dean BR, Antman KH, et al. The role of cytologic evaluation of pleural fluid in the diagnosis or malignant mesothelioma. Chest 1997;111:106–9.

49. Attanoos RL, Gibbs AR. The comparative accuracy of different pleural biopsy techniques in the diagnosis of malignant mesothelioma. Histopathology 2008;53:340–4.

50. Benamore RE, Scott K, Richards CJ, et al. Image-guided pleural biopsy: diagnostic yield and complications. Clin Radiol 2006;61:700–5.

51. Prabhu VG, Narasimhan R. The role of pleuroscopy in undiagnosed exudative pleural effusion. Lung India 2012;29(2):128–30.

52. Blanc FX, Atassi K, Bignon J, et al. Diagnostic value of medical thoracoscopy in pleural disease: a 6-year retrospective study. Chest 2002;121(5): 1677–83.

53. Boutin C, Rey F. Thoracoscopy in pleural malignant mesothelioma: a prospective study of 188 consecutive patients. Part 1: diagnosis. Cancer 1993;72: 389–93.

54. Menzies R, Charbonneau M. Thorascopy for the diagnosis of pleural disease. Ann Intern Med 1991; 114(4):271–6.

55. Harris RJ, Kavuru MS, Mehta AC, et al. The impact of thoracoscopy on the management of pleural disease. Chest 1995;107:3.

56. Swanson SJ, Herndon JE II, D'Amico TA, et al. Video-assisted thoracic surgery lobectomy: report of CALGB 39802—a prospective, multi-institution feasibility study. J Clin Oncol 2007;25(31):4993–7.

57. Jheon S, Yang HC, Cho S. Video-assisted thoracic surgery for lung cancer. Gen Thorac Cardiovasc Surg 2012;60(5):255–60.

58. Flores RM, Alam N. Video-assisted thoracic surgery lobectomy (VATS), open thoracotomy, and the robot for lung cancer. Ann Thorac Surg 2008;85(2):S710–5.

59. Czamecka K, Yasufuku K. Interventional pulmonology: focus on pulmonary diagnostics. Respirology 2012. http://dx.doi.org/10.1111/j.1440-1843.2012.02211.x.

60. Lu C, Ji Y, Shan F, et al. Solitary fibrous tumor of the pleura: an analysis of 13 cases. World J Surg 2008;32:1663–8.

61. Sung SH, Chang JW, Kim J, et al. Solitary fibrous tumors of the pleura: surgical outcome and clinical course. Ann Thorac Surg 2005;79:303–7.

62. Cardillo G, Lococo F, Carleo F, et al. Solitary fibrous tumors of the pleura. Curr Opin Pulm Med 2012;18:339–46.

63. Penel N, Amela EY, Decanter G, et al. Solitary fibrous tumors and so-called hemangiopericytoma. Sarcoma 2012;2012:1–6.

64. Steinetz C, Clarke R, Jacobs GH, et al. Localized fibrous tumors of the pleura: correlation of histopathologic, immunohistochemical and ultrastructural features. Pathol Res Pract 1990;186:344–57.

65. Cardillo G, Carbone L, Carleo F, et al. Solitary fibrous tumor of the pleura: an analysis of 110 patients treated in a single institution. Ann Thorac Surg 2009;88:1632–7.

66. Cardillo G, Facciolo F, Cavazzana A, et al. Localized (solitary) fibrous tumors of the pleura: an analysis of 55 patients. Ann Thorac Surg 2000;70:1808–12.

67. Magdeleinat P, Alifano M, Petino A, et al. Solitary fibrous tumor of the pleura: clinical characteristics, surgical treatment and outcome. Eur J Cardiothorac Surg 2002;21:1087–93.

68. Harrison-Phipps K, Nichols FC, Schleck CD, et al. Solitary fibrous tumors of the pleura: results of surgical treatment and long-term prognosis. J Thorac Cardiovasc Surg 2009;138:19–25.

69. Lahon B, Mercier O, Fadel E, et al. Solitary fibrous tumor of the pleura: outcomes of 157 complete resections in a single center. Ann Thorac Surg 2012;94(2):394–400.

70. England D, Hochholzer L, McCarthy M. Localized benign and malignant fibrous tumors of the pleura: a clinicopathologic review of 223 cases. Am J Surg Pathol 1989;13(8):640–58.

71. Jha V, Gil J, Teirstein AS. Familial solitary fibrous tumor of the pleura: a case report. Chest 2005;127:1852–4.

72. Arab WA. Solitary fibrous tumor of the pleura. Eur J Cardiothorac Surg 2012;41(3):587–97.

73. Robinson LA. Solitary fibrous tumors of the pleura. Cancer Control 2006;13:264–9.

74. Kalebi A, Hale MJ, Wong ML, et al. Surgically cured hypoglycemia secondary to pleural solitary fibrous tumour: case report and update review on the Doege-Potter syndrome. J Cardiothorac Surg 2009;18(4):45.

75. Tani Y, Tateno T, Izumiyama H, et al. Defective expression of prohormone convertase 4 and enhanced expression of insulin-like growth factor II by pleural solitary fibrous tumor causing hypoglycemia. Endocr J 2008;55(5):905–11.

76. Guo W, Xiao H, Wang R, et al. Retrospective analysis for thirty-nine patients with solitary fibrous tumor of the pleura and review of the literature. World J Surg Oncol 2011;9:134.

77. Chu X, Zhang L, Xue Z, et al. Solitary fibrous tumor of the pleura: an analysis of forty patients. J Thorac Dis 2012;4(2):146–54.

78. Mendelson DS, Meary E, Buy JN, et al. Localized fibrous pleural mesothelioma: CT findings. Clin Imaging 1991;15:105–8.

79. Ota H, Kawai H, Yagi N, et al. Successful diagnosis of diaphragmatic solitary fibrous tumor of the pleura by preoperative ultrasonography. Gen Thorac Cardiovasc Surg 2010;58:485–7.

80. Usami N, Iwano S, Yokoi K. Solitary fibrous tumor of the pleura: evaluation of the origin with 3D CT angiography. J Thorac Oncol 2007;2:1124–5.

81. Briselli M, Mark EJ, Dickersin GR. Solitary fibrous tumors of the pleura: eight new cases and review of 360 cases in the literature. Cancer 1981;47:2678–89.

82. Swanson SJ. Video-assisted thoracic surgery segmentectomy: the future of surgery for lung cancer? Ann Thorac Surg 2010;89:S2096–7.

83. Nomori H, Horio H, Fuyuno G, et al. Contacting metastasis of a fibrous tumor of the pleura. Eur J Cardiothorac Surg 1997;12:928–30.

84. Schirosi L, Lantuejoul S, Cavazza A, et al. Pleuropulmonary solitary fibrous tumors: a clinicopathologic, immunohistochemical, and molecular study of 88 cases confirming the prognostic value of de Perrot staging system and p53 expression, and evaluating the role of c-kit, BRAF, PDGRs (alpha/beta), c-met, and EGFR. Am J Surg Pathol 2008;32:1627–42.

85. Wanebo HJ, Martini N, Melamed MR, et al. Pleural mesothelioma. Cancer 1976;38:2481–8.

86. Okike N, Bernatz PE, Woolner LB. Localized mesothelioma of the pleura: benign and malignant variants. J Thorac Cardiovasc Surg 1978;75(3):363–72.

87. Takagi M, Kuwano K, Watanabe K, et al. A case of recurrence and rapid growth of pleural solitary fibrous tumor 8 years after initial surgery. Ann Thorac Cardiovasc Surg 2009;15:178–81.

88. de Perrot M, Kurt AM, Robert JH, et al. Clinical behavior of solitary fibrous tumors of the pleura. Ann Thorac Surg 1999;67:1456–9.

89. Suter M, Gebhard S, Boumghar M, et al. Localized fibrous tumor of the pleura: 15 new cases and review of the literature. Eur J Cardiothorac Surg 1998;14:453–9.

90. Veronesi G, Spaggiari L, Mazzarol G, et al. Huge malignant localized fibrous tumor of the pleura. J Cardiovasc Surg 2000;41:781–4.

91. De Pas T, Toffalorio F, Colombo P, et al. Brief report: activity of imatinib in a patient with platelet-derived-growth-factor receptor positive malignant solitary fibrous tumor of the pleura. J Thorac Oncol 2008; 3:938–41.

92. Nogales FF, Issac MA, Hardisson D, et al. Adenomatoid tumors of the uterus: an analysis of 60 cases. Int J Gynecol Pathol 2002;21:34–40.

93. Kaplan MA, Tazelaar H, Hayashi T, et al. Adenomatoid tumors of the pleura. Am J Surg Pathol 1996; 20(10):1219–23.

94. Plaza JA, Dominguez F, Suster S. Cystic adenomatoid tumor of the mediastinum. Am J Surg Pathol 2004;28(1):132–8.

95. Minato H, Nojima T, Kurose N, et al. Adenomatoid tumor of the pleura. Pathol Int 2009;59(8):567–71.

96. Murali R, Park K, Leslie KO. The pleura in health and disease. Semin Respir Crit Care Med 2010; 31(6):649–73.

97. Isaka M, Nakagawa K, Maniwa T, et al. Disseminated calcifying tumor of the pleura: review of the literature and a case report with immunohistochemical study of its histogenesis. Gen Thorac Cardiovasc Surg 2011;59(8):579–82.

98. Suh JH, Shin OR, Kim YH. Multiple calcifying fibrous pseudotumor of the pleura. J Thorac Oncol 2008;3(11):1356–8.

99. Shibata K, Yuki D, Sakata K. Multiple calcifying fibrous pseudotumors disseminated in the pleura. Ann Thorac Surg 2008;85(2):e3–5.

100. Jiang K, Nie J, Wang J, et al. Multiple calcifying fibrous pseudotumor of the bilateral pleura. Jpn J Clin Oncol 2011;41(1):130–3.

101. Pinkard NG, Wilson RW, Lawless N, et al. Calcifying fibrous pseudotumor of pleura: a report of three cases of a newly described entity involving the pleura. Am J Clin Pathol 1996;105(2):189–94.

102. Mito K, Kashima K, Daa T, et al. Multiple calcifying fibrous tumors of the pleura. Virchows Arch 2005; 446(1):78–81.

103. Jang KS, Oh YH, Han HX, et al. Calcifying fibrous pseudotumor of the pleura. Ann Thorac Surg 2004;78(6):e87–8.

104. Jayle C, Hajj-Chanine J, Allain G, et al. Pleural lipoma: a non-surgical lesion. Interact Cardiovasc Thorac Surg 2012;14(6):735–8.

105. Pinton F, Brousse D, Lemarie E, et al. Lipome pleural. Rev Mal Respir 1988;12:169–72.

106. Hayakawa M. Pleural lipoma: report of a case. Kyobu Geka 2005;58(13):1185–8.

107. Epler GR, McLoud TC, Mun CS, et al. Pleural lipoma. Diagnosis by computed tomography. Chest 1986;90:265–8.

108. Park CY, Rho JY, Yoo SM, et al. Fat-forming variant of solitary fibrous tumour of the pleura: CT findings. Br J Radiol 2011;84(1007):e203–5.

109. Yamamoto J, Shimanouchi M, Ueda Y, et al. Chest wall lipoma mimicking a well differentiated liposarcoma; report of two cases. Kyobu Geka 2012; 65(7):587–90.

110. Zidane A, Atoini F, Arsalane A, et al. Parietal pleura lipoma: a rare intrathoracic tumor. Gen Thorac Cardiovasc Surg 2011;59(5):363–6.

111. Kondoh K, Kobayashi T, Urakami T, et al. A case of pedunculated intrathoracic chest wall type lipoma. Kyobu Geka 1997;50(12):1065–8 [in Japanese].

112. Mentzel T, Fletcher CD. Lipomatous tumours of soft tissues: an update. Virchows Arch 1995;427(4): 353–63.

113. Liebow AA, Hubbell DS. Sclerosing hemangioma (histiocytoma, xanthoma) of the lung. Cancer 1956;9:53–75.

114. Devouassoux-Shisheboran M, Hayashi T, Linnoila RI, et al. A clinicopathologic study of 100 cases of pulmonary sclerosing hemangioma with immunohistochemical studies: TTF-1 is expressed in both round and surface cells, suggesting an origin from primitive respiratory epithelium. Am J Surg Pathol 2000;24(7): 906–16.

115. Keylock J, Galvin JR, Franks TJ. Sclerosing hemangioma of the lung. Arch Pathol Lab Med 2009; 133(5):820–5.

116. Chung MJ, Lee KS, Han J, et al. Pulmonary sclerosing hemangioma presenting as solitary pulmonary nodule: dynamic CT findings and histopathologic comparisons. AJR Am J Roentgenol 2006;187:430–7.

117. Bae YA, Lee KS. Cross-sectional evaluation of thoracic lymphoma. Thorac Surg Clin 2010;20: 175–86.

118. Sunil M, Reid E, Lechowicz MJ. Update on HHV-8-associated malignancies. Curr Infect Dis Rep 2010;12(2):147–54.

119. Ravikumar G, Tirumalae R, Das K. Primary pleural non-Hodgkin lymphoma in a child—an exceedingly rare disease. J Pediatr Surg 2012;47:e29–31.

120. Oikononmou A, Giatromanokaki A, Margaritis D, et al. Primary pleural lymphoma: plaque-like thickening of the pleura. Jpn J Radiol 2010;28: 62–5.

121. Barahona ML, Duenas VP, Sanchez MT, et al. Primary mucosa-associated lymphoid tissue lymphoma as a pleural mass. Br J Radiol 2011;84: e229–31.

122. Steiropoulos P, Kouliatsis G, Karpathiou G, et al. Rare cases of primary pleural Hodgkin and non-Hodgkin lymphomas. Respiration 2009;77(4): 459–63.

123. Aozasa K, Naka N, Tomita Y, et al. Angiosarcoma developing from chronic pyothorax. Mod Pathol 1994;7(9):906–11.

124. Ahmad H, Pawade J, Falk S, et al. Primary pleural lymphomas. Thorax 2003;58(10):908–9.

125. Brun V, Revel MP, Danel C, et al. Case report. Pyothorax-associated lymphoma: diagnosis at percutaneous core biopsy with CT guidance. AJR Am J Roentgenol 2003;180(4):969–71.

126. Rademaker J. Hodgkin's and non-Hodgkin's lymphomas. Radiol Clin North Am 2007;45(1):69–83.

127. Mettler TN, Cioc AM, Singleton TP, et al. Pleural primary effusion lymphoma in an elderly patient. Diagn Cytopathol 2011;40(10):903–5.

128. Moran CA, Travis WD, Rosado-de-Christenson M, et al. Thymomas presenting as pleural tumors. Report of eight cases. Am J Surg Pathol 1992; 16(2):138–44.

129. Fushimi H, Tanio Y, Kotoh K. Ectopic thymoma mimicking diffuse pleural mesothelioma: a case report. Hum Pathol 1998;29(4):409–10.

130. Shih DF, Wang JS, Tseng HH, et al. Primary pleural thymoma. Arch Pathol Lab Med 1997; 121(1):79–82.

131. Kim HS, Lee HJ, Cho SY, et al. Myasthenia gravis in ectopic thymoma presenting as pleural masses. Lung Cancer 2007;57:115–7.

132. Yamazaki K, Yoshino I, Oba T, et al. Ectopic pleural thymoma presenting as a giant mass in the thoracic cavity. Ann Thorac Surg 2007;83:315–7.

133. Kitada M, Sato K, Matsuda Y, et al. Ectopic thymoma presenting as a giant intrathoracic tumor: a case report. World J Surg Oncol 2011;9:66–9.

134. Filosso PL, Delsedime L, Cristofori RC, et al. Ectopic pleural thymoma mimicking a giant solitary fibrous tumour of the pleura. Interact Cardiovasc Thorac Surg 2012;15(5):930–2.

135. Attanoos RL, Galateau-Salle F, Gibbs AR, et al. Primary thymic epithelial tumours of the pleura mimicking malignant mesothelioma. Histopathology 2002;41(1):42–9.

136. Reid M, Potzger T, Braune N, et al. Cytoreductive surgery and hyperthermic intrathoracic chemotherapy perfusion for malignant pleural tumours: perioperative management and clinical experience. Eur J Cardiothorac Surg 2012. [Epub ahead of print].

137. Parikh M, Samujh R, Kanojia RP, et al. Peripheral primitive neuroectodermal tumor of the chest wall in childhood: clinico-pathological significance, management and literature review. Chang Gung Med J 2011;34(2):213–7.

138. Pinto A, Dickman P, Parham D. Pathobiologic markers of the Ewing sarcoma family of tumors: state of the art and prediction of behaviour. Sarcoma 2011;2011:856190.

139. Askin FB, Rosai J, Sibley RK, et al. Malignant small cell tumor of the thoracopulmonary region in childhood: a distinctive clinicopathologic entity of uncertain histogenesis. Cancer 1979;43(6):2438–51.

140. Alhariqi BA, Alamri NF. Peripheral primitive neuroectodermal tumor of the pleura in a 41-year-old female. Saudi Med J 2012;33(7):791–3.

141. Fink M, Salibury J, Gishen P. Askin tumor: three case histories and a review of the literature. Eur J Radiol 1992;14:178–80.

142. Saifuddin A, Robertson RJ, Smith SE. The radiology of Askin tumours. Clin Radiol 1991;43:19–23.

143. Winer-Muram HT, Kauffman WM, Gronemeyer SA, et al. Primitive neuroectodermal tumors of the chest wall (Askin tumors): CT and MRI findings. AJR Am J Roentgenol 1993;161(2):265–8.

144. Faubert C, Inniger R. MRI and pathological findings in two cases of Askin tumors. Neuroradiology 1991;33(3):277–81.

145. Shamberger RC, LaQuaglia MP, Gebhardt MC, et al. Ewing sarcoma/primitive neuroectodermal tumor of the chest wall: impact of initial versus delayed resection on tumor margins, survival, and use of radiation therapy. Ann Surg 2003;238(4):563–7.

146. Contesso G, Llombart-Bosch A, Terrier P, et al. Does malignant small round cell tumor of the thoracopulmonary region (Askin tumor) constitute a clinicopathologic entity? An analysis of 30 cases with immunohistochemical and electron-microscopic support treated at the Institute Gustave Roussy. Cancer 1992;69(4):1012–20.

147. Steiner GC, Graham S, Lewis MM. Malignant round cell tumor of bone with neural differentiation (neuroectodermal tumor). Ultrastruct Pathol 1988;12(5): 505–12.

148. Cattaneo SM, Klassen KP. Letter: carcinoma of the chest wall complicating chronically draining empyema. Chest 1973;64(5):673–4.

149. Willen R, Bruce T, Dahlstrom G, et al. Squamous epithelial cancer in metaplastic pleura following extrapleural pneumothorax for pulmonary tuberculosis. Virchows Arch A Pathol Anat Histol 1976; 370(3):225–31.

150. Kotani K, Makihara S, Tada R. Squamous cell carcinoma of the chest wall in a patient with chronic empyema. Kyobu Geka 2011;64(7):549–51 [in Japanese].

151. Smith S, Opipari MI. Primary pleural melanoma. A first reported case and literature review. J Thorac Cardiovasc Surg 1978;75(6):827–31.

152. Mohanty PP, Pasricha R, Gupta A, et al. Malignant melanoma of pleura in a patient with giant congenital "bathing suit" hairy nevus. Int J Clin Oncol 2004;9(5):410–2.

153. Ost D, Joseph C, Sogoloff H, et al. Primary pulmonary melanoma: case report and literature review. Mayo Clin Proc 1999;74:62–6.

154. Jensen OA, Egedorf J. Primary malignant melanoma of the lung. Scand J Respir Dis 1967;48:127–35.

155. Um SW, Yoo CG, Lee CT, et al. Apparent primary pleural melanoma: case report and literature review. Respir Med 2003;97(5):586–7.

156. Nakano M, Ujino T, Takahara M, et al. A case of primary malignant melanoma of the pleura. Nishinihon Journal of Dermatology 2010;72(6):595–9.

157. Shameem M, Akhtar J, Baneen U, et al. Malignant melanoma presenting as an isolated pleural effusion. Monaldi Arch Chest Dis 2011;75(2):138–40.

158. Dalton WT, Zolliker AS, McCaughey WT, et al. Localized primary tumors of the pleura: an analysis of 40 cases. Cancer 1979;44(4):1465–75.

159. Rdzanek M, Fresco R, Pass HI, et al. Spindle cell tumors of the pleura: differential diagnosis. Semin Diagn Pathol 2006;23(1):44–56.

160. Lorentziadis M, Sourlas A. Primary de novo angiosarcoma of the pleura. Ann Thorac Surg 2012;93: 996–8.

161. Dainese E, Pozzi B, Milani M, et al. Primary pleural epithelioid angiosarcoma. A case report and review of the literature. Pathol Res Pract 2010; 206(6):415–9.

162. Dagli AF, Pehlivan S, Ozercan MR. Pleural liposarcoma mimicking carcinoma in pleural effusion cytology: a case report. Acta Cytol 2010;54(4): 601–4.

163. Afshar M, Kim AW, Liptay MJ, et al. A 74-year-old man with an enlarging pleural-based mass that was NOT a mesothelioma. Thorac Cardiovasc Surg 2009;57:243–9.

164. Kabiri H, Elfakir Y, Kettani F, et al. Malignant primary fibrous histiocytoma of the pleura. Rev Mal Respir 2001;18(3):319–22.

165. Zhang PJ, Livosi VA, Brooks JJ. Malignant epithelioid vascular tumors of the pleura: report of a series and literature review. Hum Pathol 2000; 31(1):29–34.

166. Alexiou C, Clelland CA, Robinson D, et al. Primary angiosarcomas of the chest wall and pleura. Eur J Cardiothorac Surg 1998;14:523–6.

167. Mayall FG, Gibbs AR. 'Pleural' and pulmonary carcinosarcomas. J Pathol 1992;167(3):305–11.

168. McCaughey WT, Dardick I, Barr JR. Angiosarcoma of serous membranes. Arch Pathol Lab Med 1983; 107(6):304–7.

169. Elsayed H, Gosney J. A massive pleural-based tumour: the challenge of diagnosis. Rev Port Pneumol 2011;17(6):275–7.

170. Takahama M, Kushbi K, Kimura M, et al. Resection of primary pleural pedunculate hemangiopericytoma. Ann Thorac Surg 2004;77(6):2210–3.

171. Jain A, Safaya R, Jagan C, et al. Extraskeletal mesenchymal chondrosarcoma of the pleura: report of a rare case. Indian J Pathol Microbiol 2011;54(1):144–6.

172. Xiong WN, Fang HJ, Xu YJ, et al. Liposarcoma of the pleura: clinical characteristics. Zhonghua Jie He He Hu Za Zhi 2007;30(5):352–4 [in Chinese].

173. Luppi G, Cesinaro AM, Zoboli A, et al. Mesenchymal chondrosarcoma of the pleura. Eur Respir J 1996;9(4):840–3.

174. Wong WW, Pluth JR, Grado GL, et al. Liposarcoma of the pleura. Mayo Clin Proc 1994;69(9):882–5.

175. Moran CA, Suster S. Primary mucoepidermoid carcinoma of the pleura: a clinicopathologica study of two cases. Am J Clin Pathol 2003;120: 381–5.

176. Roh MS, Seo JY, Hong SH. Epithelioid angiosarcoma of the pleura: a case report. J Korean Med Sci 2001;16(6):792–5.

177. El Bari S, Chelluoui M, Dafiri R. Primary pleural rhabdomyosarcoma: a case report and literature review. Eur J Radiol Extra 2010;76:e55–7.

178. Goetz SP, Robinson RA, Landas SK. Extraskeletal myxoid chondrosarcoma of the pleura. Report of a case clinically simulating mesothelioma. Am J Clin Pathol 1992;97(4):498–502.

179. Alloubi I, Boubia S, Ridai M. Liposarcoma of the pleural cavity. Thorac Cardiovasc Surg 2008; 56(7):438–9.

180. Cheng YL, Yu CP, Hsu SH, et al. Hemangiopericytoma of the pleura causing massive hemothorax. J Formos Med Assoc 2000;99(5):428–30.

181. Heyer CM, Roggenland D, Muller KM, et al. Extraskeletal mesenchymal chondrosarcoma: rare differential diagnosis of pleural calcifications. Pneumologie 2007;61(2):94–8.

182. Indolfi P, Casale F, Carli M, et al. Pleuropulmonary blastoma: management and prognosis of 11 cases. Cancer 2000;89(6):1396–401.

183. Priest JR, McDermott MB, Bhatia S, et al. Pleuropulmonary blastoma: a clinicopathologic study of 50 cases. Cancer 1997;80(1):147–61.

184. Okby NT, Travis WD. Liposarcoma of the pleural cavity: clinical and pathologic features of 4 cases with a review of the literature. Arch Pathol Lab Med 2000;124(5):699–703.

185. Kao YC, Chow JM, Wang KM, et al. Primary pleural angiosarcoma as a mimicker of mesothelioma: a case report. Diagn Pathol 2011;6:130.

186. Wilson RW, Gallateau-Salle F, Moran CA. Desmoid tumors of the pleura: a clinicopathologic mimic of localized fibrous tumor. Mod Pathol 1999;12:9–14.

187. Rais G, Raissouni S, Mouzount H, et al. Primary pleural leiomyosarcoma with rapid progression

and fatal outcome: a case report. J Med Case Rep 2012;6:101.

188. Al-Daraji WI, Salman WD, Nakhuda Y, et al. Primary smooth muscle tumor of the pleura: a clinicopathological case report with ultrastructural observations and a review of the literature. Ultrastruct Pathol 2005;29:389–98.

189. Proca D, Ross P, Pratt J, et al. Smooth muscle tumor of the pleura: a case report and review of the literature. Arch Pathol Lab Med 2000;124: 1688–92.

190. Moran CA, Suster S, Koss MN. Smooth muscle tumours presenting as pleural neoplasms. Histopathology 1995;27(3):227–34.

191. Edgebombe A, Peterson RA, Shamji FM, et al. Myopericytoma: a pleural-based spindle cell neoplasm off the beaten path. Int J Surg Pathol 2011;19(2):247–51.

192. Ayadi L, Chaabouni S, Chabchoub I, et al. Primary rhabdomyosarcoma of the pleura presenting as recurrent pneumothorax. Rev Mal Respir 2009; 26(3):333–7.

193. Hamada T, Tanimoto A, Kaido M, et al. Diffuse pleural rhabdomyosarcoma with persistent pleural effusion. Acta Pathol Jpn 1989;39(12):803–9.

194. Jiang L, Zheng H, Yi XH, et al. Diffuse myxoid malignant fibrous histiocytoma of the pleura: a case report and review of the literature. Zhonghua Jie He He Hu Za Zhi 2007;30(8):565–8 [in Chinese].

195. Kushitani K, Takeshima Y, Amatya VJ, et al. Differential diagnosis of sarcomatoid mesothelioma from true sarcoma and sarcomatoid carcinoma using immunohistochemistry. Pathol Int 2008;58: 75–83.

196. Nicholson AG, Goldstraw P, Fisher C. Synovial sarcoma of the pleura and it differentiation from other primary pleural tumours: a clinicopathological and immunohistochemical review of three cases. Histopathology 1998;33(6):508–13.

197. Gaertner E, Zeren EH, Fleming MV, et al. Biphasic synovial sarcoma arising in the pleural cavity: a clinicopathologic study of five cases. Am J Surg Pathol 1996;20(1):36–45.

198. Hartel PH, Fanburg-Smith JC, Frazier AA, et al. Primary pulmonary and mediastinal synovial sarcoma: a clinicopathologic study of 60 cases and comparison with five prior series. Mod Pathol 2007;20(7):760–9.

199. Matono R, Maruyama R, Ide S, et al. Extraskeletal osteosarcoma of the pleura: a case report. Gen Thorac Cardiovasc Surg 2008;56:180–2.

200. Chandak P, Hunt I, Rawlins R, et al. Bone or pleura? Primary pleural osteosarcoma. J Thorac Cardiovasc Surg 2007;133:587–8.

201. Kim L, Yoon YH, Choi SJ, et al. Hyalinizing spindle cell tumor with giant rosettes arising in the lung:

report of a case with FUS-CREB3L2 fusion transcripts. Pathol Int 2007;57:153–7.

202. Nishio J, Iwasaki H, Nabeshima K, et al. Cytogenetics and molecular genetics of myxoid soft-tissue sarcomas. Genet Res Int 2011;2011:497148.

203. Vernon SE, Bejarano PA. Low-grade fibromyxoid sarcoma: a brief review. Arch Pathol Lab Med 2006;130(9):1358–60.

204. Meyerson SL, D'Amico TA. Intrathoracic desmoid tumor: brief report and review of literature. J Thorac Oncol 2008;3(6):656–9.

205. Bocchino M, Barra E, Lassandro F, et al. Primary pleural haemangioendothelioma in an Italian female patient: a case report and review of the literature. Monaldi Arch Chest Dis 2010;73(3):135–9.

206. Marquez-Medina D, Samame-Perezvargas JC, Tuset-DerAbrain N, et al. Pleural epithelioid hemangioendothelioma in an elderly patient. A case report and review of the literature. Lung Cancer 2011;73(1):116–9.

207. Saqi A, Nisbet L, Gagneja P, et al. Primary pleural epithelioid hemangioendothelioma with rhabdoid phenotype: report and review of the literature. Diagn Cytopathol 2007;35(4):203–8.

208. Al-Shraim M, Mahboub B, Neligan PC, et al. Primary pleural epithelioid haemangioendothelioma with metastases to the skin. A case report and literature review. J Clin Pathol 2005;58(1):107–9.

209. Klebe S, Mahar A, Henderson DW, et al. Malignant mesothelioma with heterologous elements: clinicopathological correlation of 27 cases and literature review. Mod Pathol 2008;21(9):1084–94.

210. Ng SB, Ahmed Q, Tien SL, et al. Primary pleural synovial sarcoma. A case report and review of the literature. Arch Pathol Lab Med 2003;127(1): 85–90.

211. Hill DA, Ivanovich J, Priest JR, et al. DICER1 mutations in familial pleuropulmonary blastoma. Science 2009;325(5943):965.

212. Kusafuka T, Kuroda S, Inoue M, et al. P53 gene mutations in pleuropulmonary blastomas. Pediatr Hematol Oncol 2002;19(2):117–28.

213. Syed S, Haque AK, Hawkins HK, et al. Desmoplastic small round cell tumor of the lung. Arch Pathol Lab Med 2002;126(10):1226–8.

214. Parkash V, Gerald WL, Parma A, et al. Desmoplastic small round cell tumor of the pleura. Am J Surg Pathol 1995;19(6):659–65.

215. Bian Y, Jordan AG, Rupp M, et al. Effusion cytology of desmoplastic small round cell tumor of the pleural. A case report. Acta Cytol 1993;37(1): 77–82.

216. Karavitakis EM, Moschovi M, Stefanaki K, et al. Desmoplatic small round cell tumor of the pleura. Pediatr Blood Cancer 2007;49(3):335–8.

217. Izzillo R, Lopez K, Perret C, et al. Massive benign pleural schwannoma. J Radiol 1999;80(8):866–8.

218. Morimoto J, Nakajima T, Lizasa T, et al. Successful resection of schwannoma from an intercostal nerve causing bloody pleural effusion: report of a case. Surg Today 2011;41(7):989–91.

219. Ozaki S, Miyata Y, Arita M, et al. Chest wall schwannoma associated with neurofibromatosis 2—a case report. Hiroshima J Med Sci 2004; 53(3–4):47–50.

220. Morbidini-Gaffney S, Alpert TE, Hatoum GF, et al. Benign pleural schwannoma secondary to radiotherapy for Hodgkin disease. Am J Clin Oncol 2005;28(6):640–1.

Index

Note: Page numbers of article titles are in **boldface** type.

Clin Chest Med 34 (2013) 137–141
http://dx.doi.org/10.1016/S0272-5231(13)00010-5
0272-5231/13/$ – see front matter © 2013 Elsevier Inc. All rights reserved.

chestmed.theclinics.com

Moving?

Make sure your subscription moves with you!

To notify us of your new address, find your **Clinics Account Number** (located on your mailing label above your name), and contact customer service at:

Email: journalscustomerservice-usa@elsevier.com

800-654-2452 (subscribers in the U.S. & Canada)
314-447-8871 (subscribers outside of the U.S. & Canada)

Fax number: 314-447-8029

Elsevier Health Sciences Division
Subscription Customer Service
3251 Riverport Lane
Maryland Heights, MO 63043

ELSEVIER

Moving?

Make sure your subscription
moves with you!

To notify us of your new address, find your **Clinics Account Number** (located on your mailing label above your name), and contact customer service at:

Email: journalscustomerservice-usa@elsevier.com

800-654-2452 (subscribers in the U.S. & Canada)
314-447-8871 (subscribers outside of the U.S. & Canada)

Fax number: 314-447-8029

Elsevier Health Sciences Division
Subscription Customer Service
3251 Riverport Lane
Maryland Heights, MO 63043

*To ensure uninterrupted delivery of your subscription, please notify us at least 4 weeks in advance of move.